Dementia Care in Nursing

Sue Barker
with Michele Board

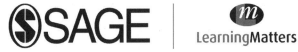

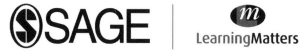

Learning Matters
An imprint of SAGE Publications Ltd
1 Oliver's Yard
55 City Road
London EC1Y 1SP

SAGE Publications Inc.
2455 Teller Road
Thousand Oaks, California 91320

SAGE Publications India Pvt Ltd
B 1/I 1 Mohan Cooperative Industrial Area
Mathura Road
New Delhi 110 044

SAGE Publications Asia-Pacific Pte Ltd
3 Church Street
#10–04 Samsung Hub
Singapore 049483

Editor: Becky Taylor
Development editor: Caroline Sheldrick
Copy-editor: Amanda Crook
Production controller: Chris Marke
Project management: Diana Chambers
Marketing manager: Tamara Navaratnam
Cover design: Toucan Design Ltd
Typeset by: Kelly Winter
Printed by: MPG Books Group, Bodmin, Cornwall

Library of Congress Control Number: 2012936252

British Library Cataloguing in Publication data

A catalogue record for this book is available from the British Library

ISBN 978 0 85725 873 1 (cloth)
ISBN 978 0 85725 801 4 (paper)

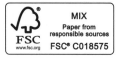

MIX
Paper from
responsible sources
FSC
www.fsc.org
FSC® C018575

Contents

Foreword

Terry Pratchett, the well-known author who has publically discussed his own early onset Alzheimer's disease, has said:

> *The first step is to talk about dementia because it's a fact, well established in folklore, that if we are to kill the demon then first we have to say its name . . . Names have power like the word Alzheimer's; it terrorizes us. It has the power over us. When we are prepared to discuss it aloud we might have power over it. There should be no shame in having it yet people feel ashamed and people don't talk about it.*
> (Alzheimer's Society, 2008a, p8)

This extremely well-written book will enable nurses not only to talk about it but also to act and care for those with dementia from a sound, knowledgeable basis that takes into account the many factors – physical, psychological and sociological – that impact on this distressing condition. Statistics about dementia feature more and more in the news. It is predicted that dementia in older people worldwide will experience an exponential rise in future years, yet more money is spent on cancer. Currently, there are 35.6 million people worldwide who experience dementia, a figure estimated to rise to 65.7 million by 2030 and 115.4 million by 2050. As nurses, we are in a key position to take on this challenge as we have close relationships with those in need of care.

Dignity and nutrition continue to be of concern in current NHS hospitals, as demonstrated in the Care Quality Commission report (2011), which identified that 50 per cent of hospitals were not providing adequate nutrition and dignity for older people. The authors, Sue Barker and Michele Board, have written a text that delves into all the aspects of nursing care that a 21st-century nurse needs to know to provide the highest standards of care for patients with dementia. They cover fundamentals, in nursing models of care, that includes compassion and caring, as well as person-centred care, and introduce a new model: humanising care (Todres et al., 2009).

The book deals with attitudes, culture and spirituality; personality and lifelong development; and assessment from a nursing perspective. Practical advice on how to manage dementia in an acute setting, including physical and psychological health, is clearly provided. All aspects of the phases of caring are covered and a very relevant final chapter on ethics and legal aspects considers issues of consent and management of complex legal scenarios and the protection of the vulnerable. The level of detail and evidence-base information in this text ensures this is one of the most readable and informative texts available on this challenging and increasingly significant condition.

Dr Shirley Bach
Series Editor

Acknowledgements

We would like to thank our colleagues and the staff at Learning Matters who have supported us in our writing. We would, though, especially like to express our appreciation for all those we have worked alongside in our caring roles. While we have endeavoured to use ourselves to show care and support others, we have felt honoured to be part of their lives. Thank you to the people who have shared their lives with us and inspired our case studies. We have met some exceptional people and feel humbled.

The authors and publisher would like to thank:

The Alzheimer's Society for the data, taken from their website (www.alz.co.uk), used in Table 1.2; royalties from the sale of this book will be donated to the Alzheimer's Society;

The Open University Press for material used in Tables 3.1 and 3.2, from Kitwood, T. (1997) *Dementia reconsidered, the person comes first.* © Reproduced with the kind permission of Open University Press. All rights reserved.

Every effort has been made to trace all copyright holders within the book, but if any have been inadvertently overlooked, the publisher will be pleased to make the necessary arrangements at the first opportunity.

About the authors

Sue Barker has been a mental health nurse since 1985 and has had a broad range of clinical experience. She started lecturing in 1998 but continued to spend half her time in clinical practice. In 2004 she became a full-time Senior Lecturer but still holds an honorary contract with a local health care trust. She has recently been involved in developing dementia care workshops for health and social care practitioners and a new unit focused on dementia care for undergraduate mental health nursing students.

Michele Board has been an adult nurse since 1985 and has had a broad range of clinical experience with a specific focus on nursing the older person. She started lecturing in 2003 and leads units on the Essentials of Nursing Care for the undergraduate nursing programme, and specialist themed days on the nursing care of the older person. She has led the development of dementia education programmes for health and social care staff working in the NHS and the private sector. She holds an honorary contract with a local health care trust working as the senior nurse for their memory clinic.

Introduction

About this book

This book is aimed at supporting pre-registration students from all fields of nursing to meet the NMC competencies, but our desire primarily is to encourage person-centred humanised care for this vulnerable group and their families. The book is organised around the NMC (2010) domains and essential skills clusters. It has activities and case studies. These will help you engage with key concepts to develop your understanding and to encourage your ability to recognise the link between theory and practice.

Book structure

This book has eight chapters. The first offers the context in which dementia nursing care may be needed, while the second explores models of care that we feel would be useful in dementia care. Chapter 3 encourages you to think about yourself, your attitudes and beliefs, and how these may affect your care and explores how these may differ from the people who may need your care. Chapter 4 explores what it means to be a person and how that may change through the lifespan along with the experiences of the person's family. Chapters 5 and 6 consider what dementia is, how it can be assessed and what that assessment and diagnosis might mean to the person. Chapter 7 explores the breadth of care interactions between you and the person with dementia. Finally, Chapter 8 offers the legal and ethical dimensions of dementia care nursing.

Learning features

Activities

There are numerous activities throughout the book that should allow you to explore your understanding and develop your thinking around the issues raised. The interaction with the materials will facilitate your understanding and memory. Some of the activities involve reflection, and as these are personal there are no outline answers at the end of the chapter. Suggested responses for the other activities are given at the end of the relevant chapter.

Case studies

The case studies have been developed from our interactions with people with dementia and their families. Pseudonyms have been used and any identifying characteristics have been changed in line with NMC (2011) codes of conduct in order to protect the confidentiality of those involved. The names that have been used are ones we have chosen and are not people known to us, so any similarity you may see as the reader between the names used and the case studies are purely accidental.

Glossary

There is a glossary at the end of the book that provides concise definitions for some of the concepts you will have read about. In the book these are highlighted in bold text at their first use.

Chapter 1
The context of dementia care

NMC Standards for Pre-registration Nursing Education

This chapter offers the context of dementia care nursing so will not address any domain in detail, but it will provide support for all four domains of the pre-registration nursing competencies, most significantly the following:

Domain 1: Professional values

5. All nurses must fully understand the nurse's various roles, responsibilities and functions, and adapt their practice to meet the changing needs of people, groups, communities and populations.

Domain 4: Leadership, management and team working

1. All nurses must act as change agents and provide leadership through quality improvement and service development to enhance people's wellbeing and experiences of health care.

NMC Essential Skills Clusters

This chapter will support the following ESCs:

Cluster: Care, compassion and communication

1. As partners in the care process, people can trust a newly registered graduate nurse to provide collaborative care based on the highest standards, knowledge and competence.

By entry to the register:

viii. Demonstrates clinical confidence through sound knowledge, skills and understanding relevant to field.

5. People can trust the newly registered graduate nurse to engage with them in a warm, sensitive and compassionate way.

By entry to the register:

x.   Has insight into own values and how these may impact on interactions with others.

Chapter aims

On completion of this chapter you should have developed an understanding of:

* the scope and breadth of dementia;
* the importance of dignity.

Introduction

A number of countries are indicating epidemic rates of dementia. In 2010 the Alzheimer's Society sponsored a study of the global prevalence of dementia; the findings estimated that there were 35.6 million people with dementia worldwide. The study's projections were that the figure would increase to over 115 million by 2050. Most of this increase is expected to occur in the developing countries, such as China, India and countries in South Asia, as they have the fastest growing elderly populations (Alzheimer's Society, 2010a). In the UK, there are 820,000 people diagnosed with dementia, costing £23 billion per year – two times more than cancer, three times more than heart disease and four times more than stroke. Alongside these figures, expenditure on dementia research in the UK has been found to be 12 times lower than for cancer (Alzheimer's Society, 2010a). It is therefore important that nurses, as health care providers, are able to identify, organise and prepare services to support this growing care need.

The statistics may lead the casual observer to believe that dementia is a disease of old age; this is not the case. Older age is a **risk factor** in the development of dementia, but it is not the cause. Along with huge increases in the number of older people with dementia there is also a worrying increase of younger people with dementia. There are 16,000 people under the age of 65 in the UK with dementia and they are more likely to have the rarer forms. The average age of people suffering from variant Creutzfeldt-Jakob disease (a type of dementia) is 29 years old (Alzheimer's Society, 2010a). People with learning disabilities such as Down's syndrome are also more likely to develop dementia at a younger age.

This chapter will provide an initial consideration of what dementia is (it will be explored in more detail in Chapter 6). It will also consider the global demographics and responses to them along with the UK situation. Finally, it will consider the professional values that are needed to underpin nursing care. This chapter therefore provides the context and background for the rest of the chapters in the book.

What is dementia and what does it mean to you?

As a reader of this book, you are likely to be a student nurse or a nurse who wishes to gain an understanding of dementia care. It is important that as nurses we recognise our values and attitudes (Barker, 2007) as, despite the availability of robust models of nursing and care pathways, the experiences of those for whom we care will be quite different from our own, depending on our underlying ideologies. Although our culture and attitudes will be explored in Chapter 3, it is worth briefly considering our starting point. Activity 1.1 will help you begin to consider what knowledge, values and attitudes you hold now. You may recognise how they develop and change through the journey this book will take you on.

Activity 1.1   *Reflection*

Take a few minutes to think about dementia. What is it? How does it affect people?

Think of a person with dementia. What images come to your mind? What age are they? What are they wearing? How do they behave?

As this activity is based on your own reflections, there is no outline answer at the end of this chapter.

We all use generalisations to help us make sense of the world, but in a society these can easily become **stereotypes**, which can be unhelpful, and in nursing they can lead us to negatively discriminate against people in our care. When undertaking Activity 1.1 you may have found that your views are based on a societal stereotype, such as 'older people get muddled just because they are old'. As nurses we often need to challenge these assumptions.

First, how is dementia defined? The Department of Health (DH) in the UK defined dementia in their *Living well with dementia* strategy as *a syndrome which may be caused by a number of illnesses in which there is progressive decline in multiple areas of functioning, including decline in memory, reasoning, communication skills and the ability to carry out daily activities* (DH, 2009, p15). Likewise, the World Health Organization (WHO), in their publication *International classification of diseases* No. 10 (ICD-10), recognised *the chronic and progressive nature of dementia which disturbs higher cortical functioning and personal activities of daily living* (WHO, 2010).

Read the case study of Mary. Do you think she has risk factors for dementia?

Case study: Mary – Part 1

Mary is 77 years old and she has been married to Stanley, who is 80, for 44 years. Before their marriage, Mary worked as a clerical assistant and returned to work part time when all her children were in full-time education. Stanley was a teacher, but they are both now retired. They have one daughter, Margaret, who is 43, and two sons, Michael, 41, and Simon, 38. Mary and Stanley describe their marriage and family life as happy, but none of their children lives close by. Margaret lives 100 miles away with her husband and two children, Emily (16) and James (12), who has a diagnosis of Asperger's syndrome. Michael is currently overseas with his young family, and Simon, although single, finds it difficult to return to his parents regularly because of work commitments.

continued . . .

> *Mary has had very few health problems; she had a sterilisation operation at 40 years old and had only minor reactions to the menopause. About 10 years ago, at a regular health check-up, she was found to have a high cholesterol level and started taking 40mg/day of simvastatin.*

If you thought Mary was likely to have dementia, why was this? Was it due to her age? Her socio-economic group? Did you think her high cholesterol might cause dementia? If you are a child nurse or a learning disability nurse, do you think that Mary's situation is relevant to you? If not, read her situation again and think about how her health might have an impact on the group of people you usually care for.

Case study: Mary – Part 2

A few years ago Stanley was becoming irritated with Mary as she appeared to be ignoring him when he talked to her and he assumed she was no longer interested in his activities. After a while he decided that it was due to poor hearing, so if Stanley wanted Mary to know something, he made sure he repeated it loudly. Mary found this irritating. Sometimes Stanley would come home and find Mary tearful, but she would just tell him not to worry – she was being silly. When Margaret, their daughter, was informed of this, she was concerned because this was unlike her mother, but she was reassured by both her parents. At Christmas, Margaret was at her parents' home with her family and Simon, and she noticed that Mary kept getting the family's names wrong and got muddled with the order of the cooking. Again, Margaret was concerned, but everyone told her that her mother was getting older – she was expected to forget things and get muddled occasionally.

Do you think getting muddled and forgetting things is a part of normal ageing? Do you think that the family arriving for Christmas expected too much of Mary? Think of people that you have met, including members of your own family. Do those over 70 have problems with their memory and get more muddled than younger people or more than they did when they were younger?

There is evidence to suggest that the ability to think logically and solve problems (fluid intelligence) decreases with age, and this is linked to physiological changes, but the ability to use skills, knowledge and experience (crystallised intelligence) may improve. Over the age of 70, short-term memory may reduce, but non-declarative memory (unconscious memory such as skills in dressing) is usually stable. Developmental changes will be considered in more depth in Chapter 4, but it is important to recognise that there are wide variations in cognitive functioning. The question nurses need to ask is what is 'normal' for the individual, not their chronological age. Older people are not a homogeneous group (they are not all the same): for Mary, cooking Christmas dinner for her extended family may be an enjoyable and achievable activity, but for others who are 77 years old it may not.

Case study: Mary – Part 3

A few weeks after Christmas, Margaret visited her parents by herself. She found her mother to be her 'normal' self, and she was again reassured. It was a couple of months before Margaret visited home again, and when she did she was surprised to hear her father grumbling about her mother becoming lazy and ignoring him. When Margaret tried to talk to her mother about what was happening, she became tearful and said she did not know what was wrong; Stanley kept getting cross, but she did not know why. Margaret thought her mother had lost weight; she also found the house to be untidy although her mother had always been keen to have everything in its place. Mary said that now she was getting older she did not have the energy to tidy after Stanley all the time, and food did not taste the same any more. Margaret assumed that her parents were becoming less tolerant of each other and that their tastes were changing as they were ageing.

What do you think of Margaret's assumptions? Do people become less tolerant as they age? Does their sense of taste change? The psychoanalyst Sigmund Freud suggested that as people age and their bodies become able to adapt, they reduce their interactions and attitudes (Stuart-Hamilton, 2000). This can lead to older people being considered rigid in their thinking and less tolerant, but other theorists, including the psychosocial theorist Erik Erikson, would disagree with this.

Erik Erikson came from the psychoanalytic perspective of psychology; he was a student of Freud. He accepted Freud's structure of the personality, but whereas Freud identified the personality as developing during childhood, Erikson's psychosocial theory outlined the development of the person throughout the lifespan. He divided the lifespan into eight stages, and at each of these the person had to negotiate a particular crisis; if the opposing elements were balanced an ego strength or virtue would be achieved. A basic overview of this theory is given in Table 1.1.

There are differing theories of late adulthood; theories such as Freud's support a disengagement approach to later life, while other theories, such as Erikson's, promote engagement. To develop

Erikson's stage	Chronological age	Crisis	Virtue
1	0–12/18 months	Trust versus mistrust	Hope
2	12/18 months–3 years	Autonomy versus shame	Will
3	3–6 years	Initiative versus guilt	Purpose
4	6–puberty	Industry versus inferiority	Skill
5	Adolescence	Identity versus identity confusion	Fidelity
6	Young adulthood	Intimacy versus isolation	Love
7	Middle adulthood	Generativity versus stagnation	Care
8	Late adulthood	Integrity versus despair	Wisdom

Table 1.1: Erikson's eight stages of life

Source: Barker, 2007

your understanding of these theories you need to read further around the subject: see the further reading at the end of the chapter.

Moving on to consider the other assumption made by Margaret – that her mother's taste may have changed – we can find some evidence to support that, too. Physiological changes in older people – for example, reduced sensual perception, such as sight and hearing – are acknowledged (Stuart-Hamilton, 2000). It is frequently physiological changes associated with ageing that impact on psychological functioning. There may, therefore, be some evidence to support Margaret's assumptions about taste but less evidence about tolerance.

Case study: Mary – Part 4

Several months passed with no indications of any problems. Margaret then had a telephone call from her father, who sounded very distressed. He said that her mother had walked out in front of traffic and had been knocked down; she was now in hospital. When Margaret arrived at the hospital she found her mother to be bruised and confused, with a broken arm. Mary could not recognise either Margaret or Stanley. She was having problems with speaking in sentences and appeared quite agitated. When the nurses tried to help her, she hit out at them and swore at everyone. Margaret was shocked by this behaviour. Michael and Simon were contacted, and both organised to return home to see their mother and support their father.

Mary stayed in hospital for three weeks, and during this time her presentation varied from calm and compliant to confused, irritable and verbally aggressive. This was distressing for the whole family, and Michael's young children became frightened of their grandmother, who had, in the past, been loving and affectionate to them. Margaret's children Emily and James thought their grandmother had become insane and enjoyed coming to see her, especially when she swore at their mother, but when their mother became tearful in front of them they struggled with how they should feel. It was thought initially that Mary was concussed from the accident and then that she might be having transient ischemic attacks (TIAs). Blood tests, urine tests, a computerised axial tomography (CAT) scan and a magnetic resonance imaging (MRI) scan were conducted to establish what was wrong. On the basis of the results from these a psychiatric assessment was undertaken, and Mary was diagnosed with vascular dementia, which is the second most common cause of dementia (see Table 1.2). Assessment strategies will be discussed further in Chapter 5.

Those of you who thought that Mary might be diagnosed with dementia were, of course, right; this is, after all, a book about dementia. Those of you who identified the increased risk of dementia due to high cholesterol also did well, but the simvastatin should have reduced this risk. The condition of **vascular** dementia, where the blood is not getting through to adequately oxygenate the brain, can be vastly improved by the use of a medication to treat the underlying cause. On the whole, though, we do not know what causes dementia or how to cure it. As nurses, this is a huge challenge, and we are in an ideal position to support people with dementia in gaining the best quality of life available to them. We also spend more time in close relationship with people with dementia and so are in a good situation to increase others' understanding of the condition and recognise where research needs to be focused.

Those of you from the fields of learning disability or child nursing can now, perhaps, see more clearly how Mary's situation is important for you to understand. She is part of a family, and each family member has a significant impact on the others. As nurses we need not only to recognise this but also to assess the needs of family members and support them.

Types of dementia

The word 'dementia' is an umbrella term, used for a collection of diseases of the brain that are progressive and terminal in nature. All of these diseases have some similar features: they affect memory, reasoning, communication and mood, but each person's illness **trajectory** or journey will be unique. The four most common dementias are described in Table 1.2.

There are a large number of other types of dementia, and some of these, along with more in-depth descriptions of signs and symptoms of those in Table 1.2, can be found in Chapter 6.

Global impact of dementia

Studies have been and are being undertaken to assess the worldwide prevalence of dementia, but the research is fraught with methodological problems. These include the sampling and diagnostic criteria, as well as demographic and cultural issues. A good spread of studies has been found in North America, Scandinavia, Europe, Japan and Australia. Researchers in India, China and New Zealand have undertaken a few, but none has been found in other areas such as Africa and Russia (Ferri et al., 2005). Despite this, it is predicted that dementia in older people worldwide will experience an exponential rise in future years (Stephan and Brayne, 2008).

Type of dementia	Brief description
Alzheimer's disease	Most common form of dementia – 62%. Brain cells die due to chemical and structural changes.
Vascular dementia	Second most common form of dementia – 27%. Related to blockages of blood to the brain cells starving them of oxygen.
Dementia with **Lewy bodies**	Third most common type of dementia – 10%. Linked to structural changes in the nerve cells in the brain and frequently associated with Parkinson's Disease.
Fronto-temporal	This is diagnosed when most of the brain cells that die are in the frontal lobe of the brain.

Table 1.2: Four common dementias

Source: information from Alzheimer's Society website: http://alzheimers.org.uk.

Alzheimer's Disease International (ADI) conducts extensive research into the global prevalence of dementia, and the needs and experiences of people with dementia (www.alz.co.uk). It produced a report in 2009 and 2010 on the global impact of dementia. Through rigorous research it was able to provide a detailed account of current global prevalence and estimate future figures. Currently there are 35.6 million people worldwide who experience dementia, a figure estimated to rise to 65.7 million by 2030 and 115.4 million by 2050 (ADI, 2009).

Dementia is currently costing US$604 billion each year, 1 per cent of the gross domestic product (1 per cent of the value of all the goods and services produced in the world each year) (ADI, 2010). Where this money is spent depends on each country's income: low-income countries spend the money available mostly on medical care, whereas in high-income countries most of the expense is in social care. Low-income countries, such as in Latin America, South and East Asia, account for only 1 per cent of the total expenditure despite a prevalence of dementia of 14 per cent. In contrast, high-income countries such as the US and Western Europe spend 89 per cent of the global figure on 46 per cent of those with the disease (ADI, 2010).

Research funding is also an issue, as identified in the introduction; despite higher prevalence rates of dementia, more is spent on cancer research. In its report on European dementia research funding, the International Longevity Centre (ILC) Global Alliance stated that dementia care is underfunded and undervalued despite the huge need. It did recognise, though, that countries such as Germany and France are making progress (ILC Global Alliance, 2011). The ILC Global Alliance organised an international symposium on dementia in 2010 to consider the issues, challenges and required responses to this perceived crisis. The product of this was to develop the following calls for action at all levels (governmental, societal, communities, groups and individuals) to protect the rights of the person with dementia and their carers.

- Engaging in a multi-disciplinary dialogue to establish a common framework of standards on preventing, diagnosing and treating.
- Developing and implementing inter-governmental and national integrated policies and plans of action dedicated to dementia.
- Supporting increased funding by governmental and non-governmental sources of research on all aspects of dementia and associated care giving.
- Increasing the number of health care professionals trained in dementia.
- Developing awareness of dementia and education aimed at preventing dementia.
- Establishing models of care for persons with dementia.
- Encouraging civil society organisations to provide advocacy and dementia care services to persons with dementia and their caregivers.
- Providing support to those persons providing informal care to persons with dementia.
- Supporting a United Nations convention on the human rights of older persons including those with dementia.
  (ILC Global Alliance, 2010)

The International Association of Gerontology and Geriatrics organised a workshop on dementia in January 2011 in which the global issues of dementia were highlighted and discussed. Peng Du from the Renmin University of China stated that society's awareness of dementia should be increased as it appears to accept dementia is a natural consequence of ageing resulting in under-diagnosis and lack of treatment. As nurses, we are in a key position to take on this challenge as we have close relationships with those in need of care. We can seek and disseminate good experiences to influence changes in practice. Peng Du (2011) went on to state that governments need to make dementia a priority in their care planning, and to invest in research and education. Health care professionals like us need to engage with health promotion and education in this area.

As nurses we can share our knowledge and understanding with those with whom we interact – our peers, our patients and their carers. We can guide them towards accurate evidence-based information such as that on the Alzheimer's Society website. We can work with other professionals such as GPs to ensure their surgeries have information leaflets and posters on display that encourage those with problems to seek help. The most important thing we can do is to be exemplary role models to others through our relationships with people with dementia.

It is clear that dementia is a concern worldwide, but as nurses we can recognise the personal and family impact of this problem. Parry and Weiyuan (2011) highlight this in their description of the experiences of a carer in China. The carer's struggle to maintain his own well-being while caring for his wife, who has dementia, is poignant but repeated throughout the world. While dementia can be seen as a significant worldwide problem, there is reason to maintain hope, as many innovative approaches are being developed to deal with current concerns (Parry and Weiyuan, 2011). Some of these approaches will be explored in Chapter 7.

UK dementia demographics

The Office for National Statistics (ONS, 2011) identified that in 2010 deaths in England and Wales due to dementia increased by 11 per cent for men and 14 per cent for women while the death rate for other major causes of mortality (ischemic heart disease, cerebrovascular disease) decreased. Dementia now has the third highest ranking for female deaths and the eighth for men.

UK response to dementia

In 2009 the UK government published *Living well with dementia: a National Dementia Strategy* (DH, 2009) followed in 2010 by *Quality outcomes for people with dementia: building on the work of the National Dementia Strategy* (DH, 2010a). The strategy was developed from a number of previous policies, as outlined in the concept summary box.

Concept summary: policy development

In the 1990s the government developed National Service Frameworks (NSFs) in their bid to ensure parity of care across the regions, as it was acknowledged that there was what was called a 'postcode lottery' – a person's care was dependent on where they lived. In 1999 the *NSF for mental health* was published. Although this did not specifically focus on dementia, Standard 1 stated that mental health should be promoted for all, along with social inclusion

(DH, 1999). In 2000 the Audit Commission report *Forget me not* found that there was limited information and understanding of dementia diagnosis and inter-professional working (Audit Commission, 2000). Sad to say, the follow-up report in 2002 found that little had changed (Audit Commission, 2002). In 2001 the *NSF for older people* was published, and one of its eight standards focused on mental health, including dementia. Standard 7: Mental Health in Older People aimed to promote good mental health in older people and to treat and support those older people with dementia and depression. To facilitate this, the standard stated that people should have access to integrated mental health services (DH, 2001a, p90). As with the Audit Commission reports, the *NSF for older people* did not appear to improve the experiences of those with dementia or their families.

In 2005 the Care Services Improvement Partnership (CSIP) published guidance on service development for older people called *Everybody's business – integrated mental health services for older adults: a service development guide* for the Department of Health (DH, 2005). It can be seen in all these governmental documents that collaborative/integrated/interprofessional working is needed to facilitate quality care. There were a number of other influential documents that also promoted collaborative working to support people with dementia and their carers: the National Institute for Health and Clinical Excellence (NICE) and Social Care Institute for Excellence (SCIE) document (NICE and SCIE, 2006), the Dementia UK report by the Alzheimer's Society (Alzheimer's Society, 2008b). The government, building on these previous reports and recommendations, commissioned the development of the National Dementia Strategy (DH, 2009).

Why do you think the experiences of people with dementia and their families did not improve? Reading the National Dementia Strategy will give a more detailed understanding of the situation (the full reference is given in 'Further reading' at the end of the chapter and in the references list at the end of the book).

Living well with dementia: a National Dementia Strategy (DH, 2009) was developed by a Department of Health group working with a large number of organisations and people through the external reference groups, which included members of the Alzheimer's Society, Help the Aged, the Royal College of Psychiatry, Age Concern, NHS Trusts, local government, social services, as well as university academics, service users and other interested parties. The consultation on the development of this strategy involved over 4,000 individuals. The aim was to ensure improvements for people with dementia in three main areas: improved awareness; early diagnosis and intervention; and higher quality of care.

The strategy sets out 17 objectives.

1. Improving public and professional awareness and understanding.
2. Good quality early diagnosis and intervention for all.
3. Good quality information for those with diagnosed dementia.
4. Enabling easy access to care, support and advice following diagnosis.
5. Development of structured peer support and learning networks.

6. Improved community personal support services.
7. Implementing the Carer's strategy.
8. Improved quality of care for people with dementia in general hospitals.
9. Improved intermediate care for people with dementia.
10. Considering the potential for housing support, housing-related services and telecare to support people with dementia and their carers.
11. Living well with dementia in care homes.
12. Improved end of life care for people with dementia.
13. An informed and effective workforce for people with dementia.
14. A joint commissioning strategy for dementia.
15. Improved assessment and regulation of health and care services and of how systems are working for people with dementia and their carers.
16. A clear picture of research evidence and needs.
17. Effective national and regional support for implementation of the strategy.
    (DH, 2009)

These can be seen to correlate well with ILC Global Alliance (2010) recommendations.

Activity 1.2 — *Critical thinking*

The aim of the National Dementia Strategy was to improve awareness, ensure early diagnosis and intervention, and provide high-quality care. It is easy to see why it is important to improve awareness and to seek high quality of care, but why do you think early diagnosis and treatment is an aim?

An outline answer is given at the end of the chapter.

Along with this strategy the government produced an implementation plan that was quickly superseded by *Quality outcomes for people with dementia: building on the work of the National Dementia Strategy* (DH, 2010a). This was developed to ensure a closer fit between the strategy and the new vision for health and care as found in the White Paper *Equity and excellence: liberating the NHS* (DH, 2010b) and *Transparency in outcomes: a framework for the NHS* (DH, 2010c). Also in 2010 The National Institute for Health and Clinical Excellence published their quality outcomes for dementia (NICE, 2010). The outcomes identified in the National Dementia Strategy, the *Liberating the NHS* outcomes framework and the NICE standards all link with each other (a table showing this can be found in annex 1 of DH, 2010c).

To support these outcomes the Department of Health commissioned Skills for Care (SfC) and Skills for Health (SfH) to provide some core principles to develop the workforce. They established eight core principles in discussion with organisations, employers, people with dementia and their carers.

Principle 1   Know the early signs of dementia.
Principle 2   Early diagnosis of dementia helps people receive information, support and treatment at the earliest possible stage.

Principle 3   Communicate sensitively to support meaningful interaction.

Principle 4   Promote independence and encourage activity.

Principle 5   Recognise the signs of distress resulting from confusion and respond by diffusing a person's anxiety and supporting their understanding of the events they experience.

Principle 6   Family members and other carers are valued, respected and supported just like those they care for and are helped to gain access to dementia care advice.

Principle 7   Managers need to take responsibility to ensure members of their team are trained and well supported to meet the needs of people with dementia.

Principle 8   Work as part of a multi-agency team to support the person with dementia.
(SfC and SfH 2011, p2)

The document provides educators with guidance and examples of how to achieve each of these principles. One example is set out in the box below.

Principle 3: Communicate sensitively to support meaningful interaction

Context

Dementia may affect the person's ability to communicate and this may fluctuate from day to day. As the disease progresses it may become increasingly difficult to communication with the person.

Indicative behaviours demonstrated by the workforce.

- Always make time for people with dementia and remain patient in every situation.
- Make use of the person's past experiences and life story to support communicating with them.
- Take into account a person's usual communication skills and background culture.
- Try to keep the environment calm and as quiet as possible when communicating, allowing plenty of time to have conversations.
- Always face the person in conversation and be reassuring in your expressions, tone of voice and words, to reduce frustration.
(SfC and SfH, 2011, p8)

These principles can help to guide managers and educators in their development of the workforce, but alongside these principles, as nurses we need to recognise the experience of dementia as just one element of the person's life world. We need to respond to people with dementia with respect and compassion, so we can help them retain their dignity and feelings of self-worth.

Dignity

In 2001, the Department of Health developed the *Essence of care* document, which provided care-givers and those needing care a description of minimum expectations (DH, 2001b). In 2010 an update was published that provides 12 benchmarks. One of the benchmarks that was in the 2001 edition as well as the updated version is 'respect and dignity' (DH, 2010d). Dignity and nutrition continue to be of concern in current NHS hospitals, as demonstrated in the Care Quality Commission report (2011), which identified that 50 per cent of hospitals were not providing adequate nutrition and dignity for older people.

Activity 1.3   *Communication*

You are working on a ward where there are number of people who have a diagnosis of dementia. It is lunchtime and you notice that one of the ladies is trying to eat soup with a fork. She is managing to get very little soup into her mouth as most of it is pouring back into the dish or over the table and down her clothes.

How do you approach the lady with respect, preserving her dignity?

An outline answer is given at the end of the chapter.

The Department of Health (DH, 2010d) defines respect and dignity thus:

Respect: regard for the feelings and rights of others

Dignity: quality of being worthy of respect

The agreed person-focused outcome of this benchmark is that people experience care that is focused upon respect. There are seven factors considered in the implementation of this benchmark: attitudes and behaviours; personal world and personal identity; personal boundaries and space; communication; privacy – confidentiality; privacy – dignity and modesty; privacy – private area. The document explains poor practice and best practice along with indicators of best practice. For example in Factor 4, communication, poor practice is where *people and carers are 'communicated at'*, whereas best practice is where *people and carers experience effective communication with staff that respect their individuality*. Indicators of best practice in Factor 4 include: using the person's preferred name; actively listening; taking into consideration individual needs; and using communication aids where necessary.

The nursing professional bodies also guide nurses towards showing respect and supporting dignity. The first statement in the nurses' code of conduct provided by the Nursing and Midwifery Council (NMC, 2011) is:

Make the care of people your first concern, treating them as individuals and respecting their dignity

Treat people as individuals

1. You must treat people as individuals and respect their dignity.
2. You must not discriminate in any way against those in your care.
3. You must treat people kindly and considerately.
4. You must act as an advocate for those in your care, helping them to access relevant health and social care, information and support.

The Royal College of Nursing (2008) states that dignity is the essence of nursing care and should be at the heart of everything we do as a profession:

> *Providing dignity in care centres on three integral aspects: respect, compassion and sensitivity. In practice, this means:*
> - respecting *patients' and clients' diversity and cultural needs; their privacy – including protecting it as much as possible in large, open-plan hospital wards; and the decisions they make;*
> - *being* compassionate *when a patient or client and/or their relatives need emotional support, rather than just delivering technical nursing care;*
> - *demonstrating* sensitivity *to patients' and clients' needs, ensuring their comfort.*
> (RCN, 2008)

While the NMC and RCN statements related to dignity and respect are to be followed by all nurses in all care situations, these values are also recognised as essential in the dementia-focused documents such as the National Dementia Strategy.

Chapter summary

This chapter has considered the context of caring for people with a diagnosis of dementia. It has identified that dementia is a global concern that is growing exponentially. There are many types of dementia, which makes dementia an umbrella term. The most common type is Alzheimer's and the second most common is vascular dementia. These two types account for 97 per cent of those diagnosed with this disorder. There is a plethora of policies from the Department of Health and other interested bodies to guide the provision of care for those with dementia. All of these, along with the nurse's professional code of conduct, dictate that nurses should care for this group of people individually, showing respect and supporting dignity.

Activities: brief outline answers

Activity 1.2: Critical thinking (page 13)

The National Dementia Strategy informs us that under-diagnosis is the current norm and that early diagnosis allows people to make choices about their health and future. Early diagnosis means that plans can be put into place so that the risk of a crisis is reduced; it also means that nurses will be able to advocate for the person as they will have had the opportunity to discuss the person's wishes in advance.

Early treatment can improve the quality of life experienced by a person with dementia. It may also reduce the time at which the person needs to seek residential care. Early treatment is important for carers as well, as treatment may reduce some of the problems they experience with managing some of the emotional behavioural issues associated with dementia by reducing them or providing a care plan.

Activity 1.3: Communication (page 15)

It is initially important for the lady to see you approaching so that you do not suddenly appear at her side. Smile at her and introduce yourself, including your role: for example, 'Hello. I am Sue and I am one of the nurses on the ward today.' Ask if you can sit beside her; if she agrees, sit down beside her so you are both on the same level. Remember that she may prefer to drop some soup and clear up afterwards and maintain her independence rather than be helped. You need to respect her wishes. Any background information on her personality will be helpful: for example, whether she is fiercely independent or fastidious.

You could broach the subject of your concern by asking if you can help or by stating that someone appears to have given her the wrong cutlery. You could offer her a spoon and, if she still has problem, offer to put the soup in a mug for her, which she can hold in two hands. It is important that you always seek consent so that the person has choice and control. If she becomes anxious and frustrated with the soup, you could offer to change it for something that she can more easily manage, such as food that can be picked up with a fork or fingers.

It is important to respond to her verbal and non-verbal cues to ensure that you respect her as a person, and maintain her self-esteem.

Further reading

Berk, L E (2007) *Development through the lifespan*, 4th edition. Boston, MA: Pearson Allyn, and Bacon.

This book offers an overview of the major developmental theories, including biological changes throughout the lifespan. It also considers the long-term consequences of certain developmental issues.

Department of Health (2009) *Living well with dementia: a National Dementia Strategy*. London: TSO.

This document sets out the government's current position on dementia in the UK along with an explanation of how the strategy was developed.

Useful websites

www.alz.co.uk

Alzheimer's Disease International (ADI) considers itself to be 'the global voice in dementia'. It provides information and advice but also has a strong research focus through its 10/66 team. This name stands for the fact that only 10 per cent of dementia research is being carried out in places where 66 per cent of the people with dementia live.

www.alzheimers.org.uk

The Alzheimer's Society website is a resource that offers health care professionals, students, carers and those with dementia information on all elements of dementia, its aetiology, treatment and impact on people. Access to support and research, along with information on how you can be involved, is also included.

www.iagg.info/

The website of the International Association of Gerontology and Geriatrics is an international site concerned with ageing that aims to foster initiatives, present actions and spread information.

www.who.int/mental_health/mhgap/evidence/dementia/en/

The World Health Organization has a huge website that offers information on all aspects of health throughout the world, including dementia. The web address above is to a page on dementia that provides links to diagnosis, information on treatments and issues related to carers.

Chapter 2
Models for dementia nursing care

continued . . .

By entry to the register:

xv. Works within the context of a multi-professional team and works collaboratively with other agencies when needed to enhance the care of people, communities and populations.

14. People can trust the newly registered graduate nurse to be an autonomous and confident member of the multi-disciplinary or multi-agency team and to inspire confidence in others.

By entry to the register:

vi. Actively consults and explores solutions and ideas with others to enhance care.

Chapter aims

On completion of this chapter you should have developed an understanding of:

- models for dementia care nursing;
- collaborative care;
- where dementia care is provided.

Introduction

This chapter explores the models of dementia care available to nurses and looks at the different fields of nursing in which this care may be given. It therefore provides the context and background for the care of people with dementia and along with the rest of the chapters in the book helps you to understand your role in caring for people with dementia.

Models of nursing care and their application to dementia

Caring is complex and skilful but there would appear to be a general assumption that these are skills that people possess naturally; they do not require learning.
(Barker, 2011, p46)

A **model** of nursing care offers a structure to bring together **concepts** of nursing and caring to guide practice, research and education. The concepts or ideas of nursing and caring are very similar as it is recognised by the Nursing Midwifery Council (NMC, 2011), the professional body of nurses and midwives, that the main aim of nursing is to care. These concepts or ideas include touch, hygiene, comfort, dignity and many more. It is important for you, as a student of nursing, to recognise the historical development of care models, particularly when caring for someone experiencing dementia. This will enable you to understand some of the practices you will observe in your clinical placements and why holistic care is so integral to nursing.

It has been suggested that holistic care is not being experienced in the National Health Service (NHS) and that this is demonstrated by the need for the introduction of the *Essence of care* guidance (DH, 2001b, 2010d), along with reports that nurses are *too posh to wash* (Hall, 2004). More recently nurses have been further condemned by reports that they *don't care anymore* (Phillips, 2011) and that many do not provide for the nutrition, hydration and dignity needs of patients (CQC, 2011). If we are to change these views and provide high-quality holistic care for people with dementia we need to understand not only the models available to us but also their historical development and how to implement them.

Historically, nursing has been seen as an adjunct to medicine and has adopted the biomedical model. This model offers a **linear process** for understanding **pathophysiology** or illness and is frequently used to explain **psychopathology**, mental illness, as well. It identifies the root cause of illness as disease, and if this disease is removed, the person will no longer be ill (Wade and Halligan, 2004). This model is limited for medicine given the current understanding of illness (Wade and Halligan, 2004), but it could be seen to be an even less useful model for nursing. The aim of nursing is to care and provide comfort (NMC, 2011), and while curing a disease may provide comfort, this is not always possible, particularly if we consider long-term conditions such as diabetes, motor neurone disease or schizophrenia.

As a nurse you will find you work alongside medical colleagues whose main aim is to identify the cause of the illness and attempt to ameliorate it by using a prescribed treatment. Many of the people you will be caring for will also have this expectation, and there are still many people who believe that the nurse's role is to carry out the doctor's instructions or prescription.

Since the time of Florence Nightingale (1820–1910), nursing theorists, guided by their philosophical world views, have developed a unique body of knowledge – nursing knowledge specifically to facilitate high-quality nursing care. Nightingale recognised nursing as both a science and an art and stated that it was separate and different from medicine. Her philosophy developed from her spirituality, her nursing experience and her caring concern for others, and continues to influence nurses today.

One of the early and influential nursing theorists was Virginia Henderson; her first book was published in 1955. The definition of nursing in this book, along with the 14 basic needs and levels of nurse–patient relationships, correlates well with Nightingale's philosophy and more recent theories and models. Henderson wrote that nursing is assisting individuals, when they needed it, to undertake activities that they would choose to undertake, if able, to maintain health, recovery or a 'peaceful death'. The goal of nursing is to facilitate a person achieving independence in these activities (Parker, 2001).

A number of caring theories related to nursing developed in the late twentieth century (1970s: Madeleine Leininger and Jean Watson; 1980s: Simone Roach; 1990s: Anne Boykin and Sarvina Schoenhofer). These theories originated from differing philosophical viewpoints, but they all imply that nursing care is humanistic in nature and involves *attitudes and values on the one hand and activities on the other* (McCance et al., 1999, p1392).

Take a few minutes to consider your philosophy of care.

- Do you think caring is natural – an ability someone is born with?
- Do you think nursing is a vocation – something you are 'called' to do?
- Do you think the biomedical approach is the best one to use when caring for a person with dementia?
- Do spirituality and/or sexuality have a part to play in your care or people's needs?

As this activity is based on your own reflections, there is no outline answer at the end of the chapter.

Simone Roach, in the 1980s, identified that it is not only nurses who provide care, as caring can be found in many areas such as family life, social care, voluntary organisations and, of course, other health professions, but that nursing care is unique. Nursing care is unique because it is generally more physically and psychologically intimate than other types of care. Roach generated the five 'C's of nursing care: *compassion, competence, confidence, conscience* and *commitment* (McCance et al., 1999, p1391). While compassion and conscience might be 'natural' attributes of most people, competence, confidence and commitment take effort to develop. Therefore, nurses need to put effort into, and be committed to, learning how to be competent in their care and through their competence feel and generate confidence. These and other nursing theorists developed a number of nursing models to offer structure to their compassion, commitment, competence, conscience and confidence.

Most of these nursing models were developed to guide nurses to ensure holistic individual nursing care. Despite this, many people with a diagnosis of dementia were still cared for using a bio-medical model.

Person-centred care

Tom Kitwood, a clinical psychologist, with his colleague Kathleen Bredin, changed the focus of care for people experiencing dementia. Given the **organic** nature of the disease, in the past care had been provided in line with a biomedical approach. Kitwood, though, developed an approach that he labelled person-centred care (Kitwood and Bredin, 1992; Kitwood, 1993). Person-centred care is about caring for the person as an individual, responding to their actual needs, not assuming their needs will follow set criteria. Kitwood's approach offers all health care professionals a way to care for people with dementia.

More recently, nursing has provided a model for working with people who have dementia. Nolan et al. (2004) developed the relationship-centred care model called the senses framework. This assumes that the nurse is in a relationship with the person with dementia and their family, forming a triad. Nolan et al. suggest that the person cannot be fully understood outside their social/

relational context. They suggest that each of those in the relationship – the person, the family carer and the nurse – need to experience relationships that promote six senses: security, belonging, continuity, purpose, achievement and significance.

Whether you see yourself as part of a 'triad' in nursing people with dementia, or working with a unique and distinct individual, the idea of the six senses may be very useful. There are links between Erikson's virtues (see Chapter 1), Maslow's hierarchy of needs (see Chapter 7), Kitwood's outline of the needs of the person with dementia and the senses in Nolan et al.'s model, and these are summarised in Table 2.1.

Kitwood's person-centred, existential approach and Nolan's relational, social approach appear to lie quite comfortably with the humanist/existential (Maslow) and psychosocial (Erikson) theories of the person.

In 2009 Les Todres, a clinical psychologist, Kathleen Galvin, a nurse, and Immy Holloway, a social scientist, brought together the humanistic, social and spiritual into organised care, found in the nursing models and care pathways, through a process of 'humanising care'. Their work has built on the early nursing theories and is consistent with the dementia care models of the person-centred approach by Kitwood and the senses framework of Nolan et al. (2004). Todres et al.'s (2009) conceptual framework proposes a continuum of humanising to dehumanising, but they suggest that most care is somewhere on this continuum rather than at one of the poles. They emphasise the need to treat people as individual human beings, respecting all aspects of the person.

Erikson's virtues	Maslow's needs	Kitwood's needs	Nolan et al.'s senses
Hope		Attachment	Continuity
	Safety/ physiological		Security
Care	Belonging	Inclusion	Belonging
Purpose	Cognitive	Occupation	Purpose
Fidelity/will	Esteem	Identity	
Love	Love	Love	
Wisdom	Aesthetic	Comfort	Significance
Skill	Self-actualisation		Achievement

Table 2.1: Comparison of needs, virtues and senses

Theory summary: humanisation of care

Todres et al. (2009) offer the following as forms of humanisation of care that you can apply to your care of people with dementia.

Insiderness
a person's subjectivity – their personal inside view of the world. Humanised care is care in which you acknowledge this and are respectful of the person's **perceptual world**.

Agency
the ability of a person to make and be responsible for their own decisions/choices. To offer humanised care you should facilitate the person's individuality, ensuring they can make their own choices.

Uniqueness
the differences between people; the people we care for are more than the sum of their parts. They are different from others and therefore you should not expect everyone with dementia to behave the same or want the same things.

Togetherness
existing in relationship with others; isolation is a huge problem for people with dementia and those who care for them. To humanise your care you need to recognise that being with family and friends is important and consider how you can facilitate this in negotiation with them.

Sense-making
our need and ability to find meaning and patterns in our world. For some this involves organised worship. To humanise your care you need to consider how your sense of the world impacts on others and how you can help them make sense of what is happening to them.

Personal journey
our lifespan development; we develop, grow and change as we move along our life line. Our individual journeys are different and we have our own goals. As a nurse you should find out the goals that people you care for have so that you can enhance their ability to achieve them.

Sense of place
our sense of belonging, our experience of being at home. When you are caring for someone with dementia it may be in their home where they feel they belong and are comfortable, but sometimes you need to organise the place they have to be (hospital, nursing home, hospice) into somewhere they can experience this. This might include personal belongings, pets or people.

Embodiment
our experience of living, our perceptions, feelings and interactions. The experiences, perception, interactions and feelings of a person with dementia should not be denied or denigrated: they are what they say they are. As a nurse you should listen to the person's expression of these and try to address any needs that occur due to them.

Theory summary: dehumanising care

Todres et al. (2009) set out the following forms of dehumanisation of care.

Objectification	This could be where you ignore or deny the person's subjective experience: for example, they state that they are disturbed at night by people banging their front gate, but you ignore this.
Passivity	This could occur by you making choices/decisions on behalf of the person because of their dementia; they then become passive by accepting your authority.
Homogenisation	This is where you expect all people with dementia to behave, think, and feel the same, and you therefore treat them the same.
Isolation	This could be where you restrict a person's social engagement opportunities due their dementia – for example, restrictive visiting, excluded access to social groups or facilities.
Loss of meaning	This could occur intentionally or unintentionally when you ignore confusion or expressed loss of meaning or make changes without explaining adequately.
Loss of personal journey	This can occur through lack of recognition of the person's goals, hopes and expectations that, despite the lack of optimal health, may still be achieved. For example, the person with dementia might like to go out to a restaurant for a meal, but you deny this because of their dementia.
Dislocation	This could occur if the person needs to move to a different care location such as a nursing home, or their condition deteriorates and the impact of this is not addressed.
Reductionist body	This could occur if a person's expressions of pain or discomfort are dismissed because it is assumed that all their expressions relate to their dementia.

A humanising agenda can be seen in the acceptance and development of innovative approaches to dementia care, which will be explored in Chapter 7. It does not aim to replace the care pathways and models that nurses are currently using, but can offer nurses a way to use them thoughtfully in a person-centred, human way.

Kitwood's reconsideration of dementia care (1997) and Nolan et al.'s senses framework can be seen to have many similarities with the humanisation of care. Todres et al. (2009) would guide the nurse to facilitate fulfilment of these needs and senses using a humanising approach. Using the case study of Karl, Activity 2.2 offers you the opportunity to consider how you might incorporate a humanising approach in your nursing care.

Case study: Karl

Karl is a 54-year-old man. He works as a technical writer for a large software company. He has two children (Cheryl, 19, and Kyle, 15), and his wife works full time as a librarian in the local secondary school. He has recently been diagnosed with dementia after a number of other conditions had been ruled out. At the moment this is only having a limited impact on his work because of his own checking processes and quality assurance mechanisms. His employers have been informed and are supportive of him remaining at work, but he has weekly meetings with his manager. It has, though, affected his relationship with his family dramatically.

His wife now monitors all he does closely; she no longer accepts his opinion and makes all his decisions for him, including what he wears to work. She is anxious when he drives the car and will not let him drive when she is in the car. His son, who lives at home, speaks to him slowly and loudly and no longer seeks his advice with homework. His daughter has stopped telephoning him from university.

Activity 2.2   *Critical thinking*

Consider the case study of Karl. Which experiences might be considered dehumanising, and how might you change these to be more humanising?

An outline answer is given at the end of the chapter.

In Activity 2.2 an exploration of Karl's situation demonstrates that a humanised approach is an essential part of your nursing care of a person with dementia, but as nurses we do not work in isolation. It is in the best interests of those we care for to work collaboratively with other professionals, agencies, carers and the person with the diagnosis.

Collaborative care

Collaboration or collaborative practice is *a relationship between two or more people, groups or organisations working together to define and achieve a common purpose* (Hornby and Atkins, 2000, p7). Based on this definition and the theories of caring above, collaborative care can be seen as people working together to support others towards the common purpose of independence in their activities of living to maintain or recover health or to achieve a peaceful death (see page 20, where this definition of care appears). Collaborative care is an important concept for nurses working with people with dementia.

Collaborative care is implicit in the National Dementia Strategy (see Chapter 1), which states the need to work closely with those with dementia, their carers, other professionals, organisations and systems. The subsequent government-funded documents (DH, 2010a; SfC and SfH, 2011) likewise promote collaborative care and have been produced in discussion with organisations, employers, people with dementia and their carers. Collaborative care is not an easy undertaking, but, with good communication and a desire to work with others in the best interests of the person with dementia, it can facilitate high-quality care.

We will now look at a number of people you may need to work with as a nurse when practising collaborative care. The list is not exhaustive as those involved in the care will depend on the person's individual needs.

Professionals

There are a number of professionals and agencies that you may need to work with in your care of a person with dementia. They could include the following.

Nurses

There will be various generic as well as specialist nurses – for example, a continence nurse – that you may need to work with. They have a similar educational background and value base to you – a holistic art and science based philosophy – and are registered with the Nursing Midwifery Council.

Doctors

As with nurses, there are a number of doctors you may need to work with – from general practitioners to specialists such as geriatricians and psychiatrists. They tend to work with a medical model and focus on diagnosis and treatment. They are registered with the General Medical Council.

Social workers

There is a generic education for social workers, but after qualifying they tend to work within specialist teams – for example, mental health. Social workers tend to focus on social problems and can be seen to use a social model of helping. They are registered with the General Social Care Council.

Physiotherapists

Physiotherapists are concerned with function and movement of the body using physical treatments. Many people with dementia struggle with mobility, stiffness and pain, and a physiotherapist can provide treatment for this and advise carers. They tend to work with a biomedical approach. They are registered with the Health Professions Council.

Occupational therapists

The role of occupational therapists is to facilitate people to be as independent as possible in their everyday tasks, whether that is paid employment or washing and eating. Occupational therapists can provide an important role in assessment of ability and support for activities for people with dementia. They are registered with the Health Professions Council.

Dieticians

Dieticians work with people to ensure they understand their nutritional needs and how to fulfil them. Fulfilment of these needs is essential to maintain good health. Dieticians may provide primary support to the individual but may also provide information and advice to nurses and carers. They tend to work with a scientific approach. They are registered with the Health Professions Council.

Psychologists

There are a number of specialisms within psychology, but those that nurses are more likely to work with are clinical psychologists and neuropsychologists. The psychologists who work in health usually use a bio-psycho-social model, but they may use any of the psychological models. They are registered to practise with the Health Professions Council, but they are chartered by the British Psychological Society.

Pharmacists

Pharmacists are experts in medication and have a scientific approach to their practice. They provide information and advice on the drugs available to people with dementia, their carers, nurses and doctors. They are registered with the General Pharmaceutical Council.

Police

The role of the police is usually to detect and prevent crime, but they fulfil a protection role as well – they can take a person to a place of safety. For example, if a member of the police force found a person inappropriately dressed and meandering dangerously close to a busy road, they could escort them to a hospital. Their approach is, though, ill defined, and they are not registered.

Statutory agencies

Statutory agencies could include:

Memory clinics

Memory problems are usually an element of dementia. At memory clinics a person's memory can be assessed, and diagnosis and treatment for memory problems can be given.

Community mental health services

These are integrated, interprofessional teams who assess and treat all types of mental health problems in the community, including dementia. The members usually include psychiatrists, mental health nurses, social workers, occupational therapists and psychologists.

Day hospitals/day centres

These can provide assessment, diagnosis and treatment for any health problem, including dementia. Some of these centres are purely for mental health problems, but others provide different types of services each day of the week. Some day centres provide social care rather than health care. The day hospitals differ from regular hospitals in that they do not provide overnight care.

General hospitals

These hospitals usually provide 24-hour care for any physical health problems. Some also provide accident and emergency services and mental health care. A person with dementia may need to access these types of care.

Specialist units

There are numerous specialist care units: neurological problem units, addiction units, dementia care units, etc. The care within them is focused on specific assessment, diagnosis and treatment needs. Most provide 24-hour care.

Social services

Social services provide for the social care of people usually through social workers, but they employ nurses and other professions as well. A person with dementia is likely to have social care needs, such as accommodation, as well as health care needs.

Carer's assessment

Any person registered as a carer for another person is entitled to a carer's needs assessment. Social services have a legal responsibility to provide this assessment and seek to address the needs of carers. As a nurse you may need to liaise with social services to initiate this assessment so that the carer can meet the care needs of the person with dementia.

Benefits/allowances

There are numerous allowances and benefits – such as disability living allowance (DLA) and attendance allowance (AA) – that the people you are caring for may be able to claim, and you may need to seek advice for them.

Resource centres

Each geographical area will have resource centres, but what is available may differ depending on the local need. Resource centres may provide information, but they may also provide aids for daily living such as tools for picking things up or aids for communication.

Continence services

Most areas' health services offer access to a continence service, usually staffed by nurses. They can provide information, support and devices to help in your care of incontinence.

Local council services

As a nurse you may need to liaise with the local council services for environmental issues such as noise control or waste disposal. They provide numerous services.

Non-statutory agencies

These could include:

Charities

There are numerous charities that could support you as a nurse working with people with dementia and their carers, including: Alzheimer's Society, Mind, Rethink, Age UK, Alcoholics Anonymous, National Society for the Prevention of Cruelty to Children, Dementia UK.

Home care services

There are a variety of these in most areas that you may need to guide people with dementia to access. They can provide services such as meals and personal care. The individual usually has to pay for these services.

Carer support groups

These can be web-based or groups set up by health, social services or charities such as the Alzheimer Society. They usually offer information, activities and support. Some offer a 'sitting' service as well. Isolation is a key problem for carers, and these groups alleviate some of this.

Self-help groups

These too can be web-based or groups set up by health, social services or charities. These groups are usually focused on a particular disorder such as dementia. They usually provide information, activities and support.

Despite the large numbers of people that could be involved in the care of a person with dementia, it is always important to negotiate primarily with the person with the diagnosis and their family. Collaborative care should occur regardless of the care environment but the people and organisations involved may differ, depending where it is given. This is further explored in Chapter 7.

Care environment

People with dementia live in the same types of accommodation as anyone else but may also reside in specialist dementia care units. There are a number of these, some of which are provided by the state (the UK government) while others are paid for by the individual or their family. Nurses from all fields meet people with dementia in any of the possible care environments. It is, though, unlikely that child nurses will undertake a caring role in an older person's hospital unit. This section will consider where and how you might come across caring for a person with dementia within your own field of practice.

Adult nursing

The focus of adult nursing is on physical health care, but it is recognised that wherever a person is cared for, their holistic health needs should be assessed and appropriate care provided. Adult nurses therefore could be providing for the physical health care needs of people with dementia in physical health settings, mental health settings, nursing and residential homes, warden-aided accommodation or the person's own home. As indicated above, this will be as part of collaborative care, and the adult nurse's role will be in accordance with their skills and the person's assessed needs. The following adult nursing scenario offers an example of care that you might be involved in undertaking in a person's own home.

Scenario: adult nursing and dementia

You work in the GP surgery (primary care) where Mrs Whittaker, aged 65, is registered as a patient. She has been attending the surgery regularly for the past five years as she developed type two diabetes, which is diet controlled, and atrial fibrillation (AF), which is treated with a beta blocker and warfarin. Since Mr Whittaker's death she has been confused about her appointment times, and her coagulation levels have been erratic. You have raised your concern with her GP, who has discussed them with Mrs Whittaker.

It is initially felt that due to her bereavement she may not have been caring for herself, her medication and diet as well as before, and that this may have resulted in her current confusion. It is agreed with Mrs Whittaker that you will visit her at home to make a more detailed assessment. At her home you find that water taps have been left turned on, there is only some mouldy bread in the refrigerator and the house is generally untidy, with piles of envelopes and chocolate bar wrappers on the floor and table.

After your visit you discuss the situation with the GP, and you both decide to call a case conference as Mrs Whittaker is recognised as a vulnerable adult. As well as you, the case conference involves the GPs from the practice, a social worker and an adult nurse from the day hospital. You discuss what you have found, and it is decided that a place at the day hospital for further assessment will be offered to Mrs Whittaker.

Mrs Whittaker is happy to go to the day hospital where she has people to talk to. The nurses and occupational therapists organise social and therapy groups for the people attending. A medication review is undertaken with a pharmacy technician, and Mrs Whittaker is provided with a dispensing box. Mrs Whittaker gradually appears less poorly and confused at the unit. Further blood tests show that her diabetes is more controlled and her coagulation rate is within the therapeutic range. It appears that Mrs Whittaker has had short-term problems associated with her bereavement. The staff at the day hospital are thinking of discharging her.

They request that you and the occupational therapist from the day hospital visit Mrs Whittaker at home to check she will be able to manage. When you arrive at her home, there is a strong, strange smell, and Mrs Whittaker is sitting in the garden in her nightwear. Inside the house you find she has placed a plastic bowl on a glowing electric ring and that the plastic has partially melted over the hob.

You make the house safe by turning the cooker off and unplugging it and leave Mrs Whittaker in the care of her neighbour while you return to the surgery to develop a crisis plan for her. At the surgery it is decided that Mrs Whittaker should be referred to specialist mental health services for assessment. Given her vulnerability, Mrs Whittaker is seen swiftly, and after some tests she is diagnosed with Alzheimer's disease.

Activity 2.3   *Team working*

- In the scenario, how many professions have you already liaised with?
- What support might be available for Mrs Whittaker?
- How can you minimise risk and facilitate the best quality care?

There is an outline answer at the end of the chapter.

As you can see in this scenario, there are a number of other people you need to work with to ensure Mrs Whittaker's safety and that her care needs are addressed. You can also see that despite working in one care environment, you need to access others to support her. As an adult nurse working with people with dementia, you need to communicate, liaise and negotiate with a variety of people in a variety of environments.

Child nursing

The focus of care of child nurses is similar to that of adult nurses, but child nurses work with a different age group (usually 0–16 years of age), which involves a unique knowledge base and unique challenges. As with other fields of nursing, child nurses need to work collaboratively to support the well-being of those experiencing dementia, whether in a primary care role or as secondary to this care. This scenario is going to consider the more common role of the child health nurse of supporting those living alongside a person with dementia, but a primary care role will be explored later in this book.

Scenario: child nursing and dementia

A social services referral has been made to the family centre where you work. A four-year-old child has been taking his clothes off, swearing intermittently with no apparent cause, taking other children's belongings and occasionally sitting in a corner crying. The nursery school has raised concerns with social services, and they have spoken to the child's mother, as the behaviours appear similar to those expressed by children after a traumatic experience. It becomes apparent in their conversation that the child has seen some of the behaviours exhibited by his grandmother and has been re-enacting some of them at nursery school. His grandmother has been living in the family home but has become disorientated, confused and at times aggressive. This is seen as deterioration in her mental state, and she has a diagnosis of fronto-temporal lobar dementia. She has now been admitted to a mental health unit for assessment and treatment.

The mother is able to visit the grandmother during nursery times, so the child is having a break from his grandmother. Despite this, the child is still exhibiting the challenging behaviour. Through your discussion with the child's mother and social worker it is decided that they will give the child a programme using a star chart for use at home and at nursery. When the child behaves in a way that is acceptable, he is to be given a star to go on his chart. Once he has collected five stars he is to be allowed to choose a reward. It is also decided that once a week you will spend some time with him, allowing him the opportunity, while playing, to talk about his grandmother and her behaviour.

---

continued . . .

At the mental health unit the grandmother's medication has been reviewed and some behaviour management interventions implemented. They now want to discharge the grandmother back to the family home.

Activity 2.4   *Critical thinking*

- Who should take part in the discharge planning to predict risks and minimise the impact of them?
- What support is available to the mother?
- What can you do in your role as a child health nurse to ensure the well-being of the child?

There is an outline answer at the end of the chapter.

While child nurses primarily provide care for infants, children and young people, this does not occur within a vacuum. Child nurses need to consider the care context and the environment in which the children that need their support are living, as this can guide the care needed and reduce the risk of future relapse.

Mental health nursing

Mental health nurses work with people regardless of their age. They engage with mothers and babies, children, adolescents, adults and older adults. They work to support recovery and well being with people with mental health problems that may be short term, for example after the birth of a baby, or with people who have long-term conditions. Mental health nurses can work in any care environment, but most people are cared for in their own homes.

Scenario: mental health nursing and dementia

Michael Bennett is a 68-year-old man who has been referred by his GP to the Older Persons Community Mental Health Team (CMHT) that you are allocated to as a student nurse. Your mentor, a community mental health nurse who specialises in working with older people, has been asked to visit Michael at home to undertake an assessment of his mental health.

The GP referral is very brief; it indicates that Michael's wife is concerned about his behaviour, but particularly his memory. The GP has undertaken the standard blood and urine tests but these have indicated no significant abnormalities. The GP is unsure whether the changes noticed by Michael's wife are due to a reactive depression due to the recent death of both of his parents or due to dementia.

A visit is arranged, and permission is given for you to take part in the assessment. Michael explains that he does not believe your visit is necessary but he has agreed to speak to you as his wife is concerned. He says that his memory is not as good as it used to be and admits he has got lost going to the shops a few times, but he

continued . . .

states that this is what you expect when you get older. He also agrees that he does not enjoy things as much as he used to and that his appetite and sleep have not been good.

Michael's wife appears tired and anxious, She explains – frequently looking at Michael – that gradually since his retirement at 64 his memory has become worse, and that he no longer does the gardening or odd jobs around the house or attends the rotary club of which he is a member. He has got lost when going to the shops and they have had to call the police to find their car, which they assumed was stolen when Michael took it out and could not find it. He has also rung the police on a few occasions at night as he has thought they were being burgled.

Michael sits impassively while his wife is talking, and at the end he says that he has no recollection of these things but does not believe his wife would lie to him. He said he does get angry with her and shouts at her when she says these things, which is unlike him. His wife agrees that he is quite a philosophical man and never shouted at their children.

You undertake a mini mental state examination (MMSE) (Folstein et al., 1975), an older person's risk assessment provided by the local NHS Trust and a depression inventory. Michael scores 20 on the MMSE (see Chapter 5), and he is assessed as at moderate risk of being vulnerable to others and at some risk of harm to others. You also assess him to have mild depression.

Given the information you have gained from Michael and his wife it seems likely he has dementia, but you recognise this will need further exploration.

Activity 2.5 — *Critical thinking*

- Who has been involved supporting Michael's well-being so far?
- Who else and what groups/organisations might be able to offer support to Michael and his wife?
- What advice would you give to Michael and his wife while they await a formal diagnosis?

There is an outline answer at the end of the chapter.

Mental health nurses work with people with all types of dementia, but the scenario of Michael and his wife is a fairly common one. There are many sources of support that Michael and his wife will be able to access. Key concerns for the mental health nurse at this stage are for Michael and his wife to gain an accurate diagnosis and assessment for medication, to gain information that they can understand and to receive emotional support.

Learning disability nursing

Learning disability nurses work with people, regardless of age, who have significant problems with learning. This is frequently due to congenital or inherited problems, but may also be due to neurological problems such as epilepsy. They work to protect the well-being and social inclusion of this vulnerable group. Learning disability nurses, like mental health nurses, work within all the diverse care environments. The learning disability nurse scenario offers one care context, but it can be seen that although they are caring for the woman in her own home, what is recognised as home changes for her.

Scenario: learning disability nursing and dementia

Stacey Roberts, 42, lives in a small shared house near the centre of the town in which she grew up. When she moved there from her parents' home at the age of 28, the integrated health and social care learning disability team initially visited once a week to ensure she was coping with her day-to-day requirements.

Stacey enjoyed having independence and her own space but also others to talk to and watch television with in the shared sitting room. Initially, she needed a lot of support with managing her finances, but she gradually managed to be independent in this as well. Despite her new independent lifestyle, she still visited her parents once a week for a family meal.

The learning disability team continued to visit the house in which Stacey lived but only when invited by the residents. The four residents found each other's company reassuring and comforting and rarely asked for assistance from the team.

However, the team has received a telephone call from one of the residents, who sounds quite distressed, asking for someone to visit. When you, as a learning disabilities nurse, arrive at the house, you find Stacey tearful, with one of the female residents shouting at the others with her arm around Stacey. The residents tell you that Stacey has been quite tearful and has been going into the other residents' rooms at night. Stacey does not remember doing this. The female resident who is comforting Stacey says that they have been concerned and that she has taken Stacey to see the GP. The GP did some tests, but said that there was nothing wrong with her and that you should be contacted.

When you talk to Stacey you find that she is a little confused and disorientated and that she has a faint smell of stale urine. You contact the GP surgery and arrange to escort Stacey to another appointment. Your concern is that Stacey may have an infection and that the GP has not heard what Stacey has been trying to say because of her current health problem and her learning disability. When Stacey and you meet with the GP you find that the GP has undertaken blood and urine tests and found no abnormalities. Given Stacey's level of confusion and distress, together you agree that Stacey should have some psychological tests rather than a computerised axial tomography (CAT) or magnetic resonance imaging (MRI) as she might find this too stressful.

The psychologist undertakes some tests with Stacey with you present so that you can reassure her. It is identified that Stacey has significant memory loss, reduced problem-solving abilities and rapid mood swings. It is concluded that Stacey has early onset dementia probably related to her genetic disorder of Down's syndrome.

Activity 2.6   *Critical thinking*

- Who has been involved in supporting Stacey's well-being so far?
- Who else and what groups/organisations may be able to offer support to Stacey?

continued . . .

- What immediate advice could you offer Stacey and the other residents to maintain their sense of well-being?

There is an outline answer at the end of the chapter.

The main role of a learning disability nurse is to support the independence of the people they work with through liaison, negotiation and advocacy; this can be seen in the scenario.

As can be seen, in all four of the above scenarios, for people with dementia, their families' and their carers' collaborative care is essential. It is also clear that people with dementia can live in numerous different types of accommodation – in fact, in more types than a person without dementia.

How you, as a nurse, interact and work with others depends on your knowledge, values and attitudes, and this will be further explored in Chapter 3. Take a few minutes to undertake Activity 2.7 to assess any changes that engaging with this chapter may have facilitated.

Activity 2.7   *Reflection*

Return to your thoughts from Activity 2.1 and see if your philosophy of care has changed in light of these theories of care.

As this activity is based on your own reflections, there is no outline answer at the end of this chapter.

It is hoped that this chapter has increased your knowledge, and it may have changed your attitude towards dementia. As authors it is our passionate desire that people with dementia will receive excellent care and enjoy a good quality of life. We hope that you too desire this and that we, through this book, can help you achieve it.

Chapter summary

This chapter has considered the context of caring for people with a diagnosis of dementia. The development of dementia nursing care models was considered, including the biomedical model, and it was suggested that a humanising approach offers the best-quality care. A collaborative approach to this care is essential, as it maximises the knowledge and skill available to ensure that the needs of the person, their family and carers are met. A scenario for each of the fields of nursing was described along with self-assessment activities.

Activities: brief outline answers

Activity 2.2: Critical thinking (page 25)

Dehumanising experiences	Dehumanising behaviour	Behaviour change to support humanising	Humanising experiences from changed behaviour
Objectification	Karl's wife and children no longer seek his opinion – his perceptions and views are no longer acknowledged or valued.	You could support Karl's family to return to seeking and listening to Karl's thoughts, opinions and understanding. They need to recognise that even if his perceptions are not the same as theirs, they are his and therefore significant.	**Insiderness**
Karl is experiencing passivity	Karl's wife no longer allows him to make his own decisions/choices. Karl may be experiencing passivity in regard to his weekly meetings with his manager	As a nurse working with Karl and his family you could encourage and guide his wife to support him in making his own decisions, getting them to discuss fears over risky choices. Karl could be supported by you to be assertive in these meetings by being open and honest and taking a written agenda with him to the meetings and taking notes while there.	Agency
Homogenisation	Karl's family are making assumptions about his ability based on their understanding of dementia.	You need to provide information and education for the family so that they recognise that every journey with dementia is different	**Uniqueness**

Dehumanising experiences	Dehumanising behaviour	Behaviour change to support humanising	Humanising experiences from changed behaviour
Isolation	Karl's son no longer discusses his homework with him and his daughter does not telephone him.	Either you or Karl's wife could discuss the situation with the children and educate them about their father's condition and advise them of the importance for them and him of maintaining their previous relationships as much as possible.	**Togetherness**
Loss of meaning	Karl's previous world has fallen apart with changes at work and home. His understanding of why this is happening may take many forms depending on his previous way of making sense of the world.	If Karl made sense of the world through organised religion, perhaps meeting with his spiritual leader will help him make sense of things. You could guide him to do this. It may be that sitting fishing helps him resolve the chaos endemic in our world and you could help his wife facilitate this.	Sense-making
Loss of personal journey	Karl's journey has changed and at the moment he is being given very little opportunity to achieve original goals or develop new ones.	You could discuss with Karl what he wanted to achieve, what his goals were and how he might achieve these and perhaps consider new goals that can be achieved with his new direction.	**Personal journey**

Dehumanising experiences	Dehumanising behaviour	Behaviour change to support humanising	Humanising experiences from changed behaviour
Dislocation	Karl may feel dislocated from his family and his place within it. His family are behaving towards him in significantly different ways to prior to diagnosis.	Things will be different for Karl and so he will need to develop a new sense of place. This can be facilitated by his family maintaining their contact with him and any changes that need to occur being put into place at his pace with full explanations and discussions. These may need repeating or writing down; you could support them with this.	**Sense of place**
Reductionist body	At the moment the focus of everyone Karl is significantly in contact with is on his brain disease; this is reductionist.	As Karl's nurse you need to work with him and his family to understand that Karl is still a whole person. He can still gain pleasure from activities, his senses and interactions. His expression of these should be acknowledged and respected by you and them.	**Embodiment**

Activity 2.3: Team working (page 31)

You have already liaised with five other professionals (GP, social worker, occupational therapist, pharmacy technician, day hospital nurse); you have also liaised with Mrs Whittaker's neighbour.

There are a number of support mechanisms for Mrs Whittaker if she should remain in her own home, but she could also move to warden-aided accommodation, a residential home or a nursing home. Mrs Whittaker will need further assessment in her home situation to assess if she can manage to remain there or need to move. If Mrs Whittaker is assessed as safe to remain at home at present she can be guided to gain support from: the day hospital or day centre, Older Persons CMHT, her neighbour (with Mrs Whittaker's permission), Alzheimer's Society, social services, Age UK and home care services.

To minimise risk and facilitate the best quality of care for Mrs Whittaker, you need to ensure you work collaboratively with the inter-professional team and, liaise with local agencies and her neighbour. A comprehensive assessment needs to be conducted and, as the CMHT has been involved, it may be best placed to undertake this through the Care Programme Approach (see Chapters 5 and 7). After this assessment she may return to your care, but you should be provided with a comprehensive risk assessment and identified needs.

Activity 2.4: Critical thinking (page 32)

As the grandmother has been an in-patient of a mental health unit, the team there will organise a Care Programme Approach (CPA) discharge meeting. As part of this meeting all those involved in her care should be invited. Therefore, she herself will be invited, as will her care coordinator from the CMHT, the older persons' psychiatrist and the mother, as her carer. Given the needs of the child, the children's social worker and you may be invited, and you may request to be involved. You and the children's social worker will need to inform the meeting of the possible impact of the grandmother's behaviour and distress on the child and consider how these can be managed. See Chapter 6 for more information on fronto-temporal lobar dementia. Risks could involve the grandmother misperceiving events and exhibiting what appears bizarre behaviour, such as becoming aggressive or taking her clothes off. These things are more likely to occur when the grandmother is stressed by events leading up to the misperception. You could work with the family to establish an ABC (Antecedent, Behaviour Consequence) diary in which to monitor and ameliorate these by early intervention, changing the antecedent.

Support available for the mother, the main carer for the grandmother, is multi-faceted. The care coordinator will provide support for her, but they would recommend a carer's needs assessment is undertaken by a social worker. She could access support groups from health and social care services and through organisations such as the Alzheimer's Society. She would be able to access support with the care of her child through the nursery, the family centre and social services.

In your role as a child health nurse you can help ensure the well-being of the child in a number of ways. You can provide support directly to the child as described in the scenario, but it would be in everyone's best interest if preventative measures were taken rather than these reactive ones. You could offer guidance to the mother and the nursery on how to address any concerns the child might have about the grandmother and encourage them to give the child space to talk about her. You also need to liaise with the care coordinator if you have concerns, as they will be able to offer support and guidance to you.

Activity 2.5: Critical thinking (page 33)

So far Michael has been supported mostly by his wife and to some extent by his GP.

There are a number of sources of support for Michael and his wife, including the community mental health nurse you are working with. Michael will need your initial assessment confirmed through an accurate diagnosis; this can be conducted by the psychiatrist for older people, who may also be able to support Michael's well-being by prescribing medication to help. Michael's wife will be entitled to a carer's assessment, where her support needs can be assessed and provided for; usually this is undertaken by a social worker. Attending a day centre or day hospital may be helpful to Michael as he could receive support from a number of professionals there (occupational therapists, physiotherapists, dieticians, nurses, etc.) to address his holistic needs. Michael may also find support from the rotary club he used to attend, along with a number of other recreational organisations. There are many other organisations that might support Michael and his wife, including the Alzheimer's Society, Age UK and Dementia UK.

To maximise Michael's sense of well-being, you might advise that he continues with as many of his previous activities as possible, maintains contact with friends, takes regular exercise and eats a healthy balanced diet.

All of these will give him optimal opportunities for improving his mood and his cognitive skills. You could also offer some simple suggestions for maximising his memory such as the use of diaries, calendars and electronic devices for locating things such as keys.

Activity 2.6: Critical thinking (pages 34–5)

So far, a number of people have been involved in supporting Stacey: primarily her parents, the other residents and her GP but also social services and the integrated learning disability team.

Given Stacey's current diagnosis, she will need increased support over the coming years. The integrated learning disability team will be able to offer her support with daily living activities, finances etc. Her mother and the other residents will be able to offer her psychological support, particularly emotional support. The Alzheimer's Society and organisations such as Scope are available to offer support, information and advice to people in Stacey's situation. As her problems progress, day hospitals and centres may offer support, and at some point Stacey may need support from a nursing home.

To support Stacey and the other residents while additional support for them is explored, you could suggest that they label things in a way that makes it clear what belongs to whom. For example, on each of their bedrooms they could put a picture of themselves or of something they like, not only to identify that it is their room but also to trigger recognition of them as a person to help Stacey. With Stacey's permission you will need to explain to the other residents what is happening and how they can support her. You might also suggest that they can support Stacey by helping her to understand what is happening by giving clear explanations and that they should all continue to do the things together that they used to enjoy.

Further reading

Barrett, G, Sellman, D and Thomas, J (2005) *Interprofessional working in health and social care: professional perspectives*. Basingstoke: Palgrave Macmillan.

In Part I this book offers an overview of interprofessional working and why it is necessary. In Part II it uses case studies to consider the issues of this way of working for a number of professional groups including nursing.

Department of Health (2010) *Essence of care*. London: Department of Health.

A version of this can be found on the Department of Health website. This is essential reading for student nurses as it sets out the government guidelines on minimum expectations of care in the NHS for the public.

Useful websites

http://guidance.nice.org.uk/CG42

The National Institute for Health and Clinical Excellence website provides guidance on the use of the dementia care pathway it has developed, including the use of medication.

http://shura.shu.ac.uk/280

This page on the Sheffield Hallam University website provides a report on the GRIP (*Getting research into practice*) report for the senses framework for dementia care, giving a more detailed account than is available in this book.

www.jrf.org.uk/publications/promoting-person-centred-care-front-line

Working with Stirling University, the Joseph Rowntree Foundation has developed a report on person-centred care, considering the implications for frontline workers such as yourself. This website gives access to the full report.

Chapter 3
Attitudes, culture and spirituality

NMC Standards for Pre-registration Nursing Education

This chapter will address issues within all four domains of the pre-registration nursing competencies but most significantly the following:

Domain 1: Professional values

2. All nurses must practise in a holistic, non-judgemental, caring and sensitive manner that avoids assumptions, supports social inclusion; recognises and respects individual choice; and acknowledges diversity. Where necessary, they must challenge inequality, discrimination and exclusion from access to care.

Domain 4: Leadership, management and team working

4. All nurses must be self-aware and recognise how their own values, principles and assumptions may affect their practice. They must maintain their own personal and professional development, learning from experience, through supervision, feedback, reflection and evaluation.

NMC Essential Skills Clusters

This chapter will support the following ESCs:

Cluster: Care, compassion and communication

3. People can trust the newly registered graduate nurse to respect them as individuals and strive to help them preserve their dignity at all times.

By entry to the register:

iv. Acts professionally to ensure that personal judgements, prejudices, values, attitudes and beliefs do not compromise care.

4. People can trust a newly qualified graduate nurse to engage with them and their family or carers within their cultural environments in an acceptant and anti-discriminatory manner free from harassment and exploitation.

By entry to the register:

v. Is acceptant of differing cultural traditions, beliefs, UK legal frameworks and professional ethics when planning care with people and their families and carers.

continued . . .

5. People can trust a newly registered graduate nurse to engage them in a warm, sensitive and compassionate way.

By entry to the register:

x. Has insight into own values and how these may impact on interactions with others.

Chapter aims

On completion of this chapter you should have developed an understanding of:

- your own and others' attitudes towards people with dementia;
- culture and its impact on the person and dementia care;
- how you can engage with people's spirituality to facilitate well-being.

Introduction

People with a diagnosis of dementia have been **stigmatised**, and negative attitudes have been widespread. A recent report was described in the press: *Up to three quarters of dementia sufferers remain undiagnosed due to the lingering stigma over the condition and the belief of some doctors that little can be done to help them* (Adams, 2011). This chapter will explore our attitudes and the way they are developed within a culture. It will also help you to understand what is meant by spirituality and how you can use the spiritual sense of people with dementia to help in their care.

Attitudes

Attitudes have been considered the most important concept in social psychology, and an understanding of them is of particular relevance to nursing today. **Attitudes** can be defined as the emotional, cognitive and behavioural response to the underlying beliefs and values of the person (Barker, 2007). So your attitude to people with dementia is your response to them based on your own values and beliefs. Some attitudes are expressed explicitly; others guide behaviour at an unconscious level. There is, though, some controversy over how much a person's attitudes actually guide their behaviour, as little **correlation** (similarity) has been found between what people say their attitudes are and their behaviour.

Nursing literature and our professional code of conduct encourage us to recognise the attitudes, values and beliefs that guide our actions, particularly those that influence our care. Consider what the attitudes of the nurses in Activity 3.1 might be and how this might affect their care.

Activity 3.1   *Critical thinking*

Martin and Sarah are graduate nurses and both work on a busy assessment ward. They are conscientious, caring and mindful of the evidence that underpins their practice.

Martin is an elder child. He felt loved by his parents and in turn he loved his younger brother but frequently felt responsible for him. His younger brother was quite adventurous and was a frequent visitor to the local accident and emergency department. Martin recognised the concern and distress this caused his mother. He learnt to be vigilant and managed to allow his brother to have fun at the same time as keeping him safe.

Sarah has two older brothers, of whom she is very fond and proud. She enjoyed climbing trees and playing football with them when she was young despite her mother and father wanting her to be their 'little princess'. Her two brothers achieved good qualifications at school and she had felt the need to do the same, which took quite a lot of effort for her. Sarah's parents were very proud of their children's achievements.

What sort of values and attitudes do you think Martin and Sarah might hold?

How do you think this might influence their care?

An outline answer can be found at the end of the chapter.

Although Martin and Sarah may not have recognised the reasons for their attitudes, and the values that underpin them, it is important that they develop self-awareness to ensure that their attitudes do not negatively affect the care they give.

Activity 3.2   *Reflection*

Spend a few minutes thinking about what is important to you in nursing. Look at the list of concepts in nursing below, and organise them into the most important to you at the top and the least important at the bottom. How might your choices affect your care? Try to identify one possible positive and one possible negative outcome of your preferences when you are working with people with dementia.

- Touch, including hand holding, hugging, stroking.
- The use of humour.
- Risk management.
- Care planning.
- Hygiene.
- Expressing sexuality.
- Assessment.
- Listening.
- Autonomy.

As this is a personal reflection, there is no outline answer at the end of the chapter.

It is not only a nurse's individual attitudes that affect their care, as all of us are influenced by stereotypes. Stereotypes can be useful, as they provide categories that reduce the effort our brain needs to undertake in everyday life. For example, if you find a romantic novel left behind by a visitor, you might save time by calling to the woman leaving the ward, rather than the man, to ask if it is theirs. All mental processing takes time and energy, and stereotypes can offer a short cut. The problem comes when stereotypes are used to make decisions about individuals. No one individual will fit a stereotype in every way, so using these to make decisions in our care can lead to **discrimination** and in extreme cases **social exclusion** and **abuse**. The case study of Aida will help you start to understand this problem.

Case study: Aida

Aida had worked as a nurse for 25 years, caring for people who were acutely physically unwell. It was a very busy environment that needed mental alertness, quick responses, a deep understanding of people's needs and lots of energy. Aida retired at 55 due to health problems and a few years later was diagnosed with vascular dementia. She had had a wide group of friends who had initially stayed in contact with her when she retired; they met for lunch once a month.

Aida was married with one daughter. When she was diagnosed, Aida's husband started to take over all the decision-making and always arranged for himself or their daughter to escort Aida when she left the house.

Initially, when Aida started to forget some of her friends' names and details about them, they were sympathetic, but after a few months she stopped being invited to the lunches. Her husband contacted them to ask what was happening, and one friend said they had thought that not inviting her would be the kindest thing to do, given Aida's condition. They said she would quickly forget that she used to attend, and it would be embarrassing for her if they kept having to remind her who they were. They also thought that it would reduce his workload as he would not need to escort her.

There may be a number of explanations for Aida's friends' decision, such as their embarrassment at her behaviour, along with other issues such as her husband's control and the removal of Aida's autonomy. Aida's friends and family would probably not have behaved as they did without the underlying stereotyped beliefs about dementia that are prevalent in our culture. A person with dementia is believed to be old, forgetful of recent events, non-communicative, unable to make decisions, lacking understanding and unaware of what is happening around them. All this is incorrect, and it is a problem. This stereotype is doubly problematic as the stereotype of ageing or **ageism** is also associated with it. A search through popular media will lead to a discovery of *pictures of elders with sagging bodies, dim eyes, and limited mobility, ads offering miracle cures for these 'diseases' and deceptive ads urging people to buy insurance polices for long term care* (DeMuth, 2004, p64). These, along with other societal views that older people are dependent, unsafe and incontinent, create a negative social environment for someone with dementia. As nurses we are obliged to tackle discrimination and advocate for those for whom we care; this includes raising awareness and providing health education. Read the case study of Bruno Berger and consider how you might have approached undertaking his admission.

Case study: Bruno Berger

Bruno had been admitted from his nursing care home to an older persons' unit for a few days. This was primarily to review the medication for his Parkinson's disease, as his speech and mobility had been decreasing and he had been experiencing some auditory hallucinations (hearing voices). Bruno was also becoming more confused and the Parkinson's nurse specialist was concerned. Bruno also had a diagnosis of dementia with Lewy bodies. On admission the nurse asked the person escorting him from the nursing home all the admission assessment questions, including what he liked to be called. A name band was put on his wrist without explanation, and the nurse helped him up and out of his chair. Later when he was physically examined by the doctor the nurse helped him undress and provided all the information for him.

Activity 3.3   *Critical thinking*

Reread the case study of Bruno. What assumptions do you think the unit nurse was making?

What do you think these assumptions were based on?

Do you think her actions were discriminatory?

An outline answer is given at the end of the chapter.

As nurses we need to be mindful of our attitudes and values to ensure they do not lead us to discriminate against the people for whom we care. Our attitudes are said to be primarily influenced by the values, beliefs and assumptions that we learn from our environment. Kitwood (1997) suggested that nurses and other health care professionals are caught up in certain discourses which lead to what he has labelled **malignant social psychology (MSP)**. This is where nurses, through their culture, view the person with dementia in a malignant or negative way, not through malice or intent but through immersion in this culture. Initially, Kitwood identified 10 MSP elements, but he later developed this to 17 (Kitwood, 1997), as shown in Table 3.1.

Malignancy	Examples
Treachery	The nurse manipulates the person into complying with them. For example, the person states they would like a drink, and the nurse says, *If you come with me, I will get you a drink* and then actually takes them to the bathroom.

Table 3.1: Kitwood's 17 malignancies

Source: Kitwood, 1997.

Continued

Malignancy	Examples
Disempowerment	The nurse reduces the person's ability to take control. For example, the person may be able to use a fork but the nurse only provides them with a spoon.
Infantilisation	The adult is treated as if they were a small child. For example, when the nurse is giving a person their lunch, she says, *There we go – you eat that all up like a good girl and don't spill it down yourself.*
Intimidation	This situation could be seen to occur if the nurse says to a person walking towards the door, *Don't you dare go out of that door or I will take your shoes and coat away.*
Labelling	An example could be a person noisily seeking attention and the nurse explaining to the visitor, *Oh that is just because of the dementia.*
Stigmatisation	For example, one nurse talking to another about working in a particular area states, *Oh, you don't want to work there – they are all demented down there.*
Outpacing	The nurse works at a pace that is too fast for the person – for example, giving information too quickly for them to understand.
Invalidation	For example, the person says they are unhappy, and the nurse says, *No, you're not; it is a lovely sunny day, which makes you happy.*
Banishment	For example, the person comes up to the nurse while she is sitting reading notes, and the nurse says, *No, go away. I'm too busy to deal with you now.*
Objectification	The person is treated as if they are an object. For example, the person is sitting in a wheelchair and is suddenly moved to another area without explanation.
Ignoring	For example, two nurses sit talking to each other across the person without acknowledging the person is there.
Imposition	The nurse forces the person to do something they do not want to do, such as turning the television on in the room when the person did not want to watch it.
Withholding	For example, a person requests a drink but is ignored.
Accusation	The nurse blames the person when they are unable to change the situation. For example, a drink intended for someone else is put by the side of the person, and the person drinks it as they believe it is for them.
Disruption	For example, the person is in the middle of reminiscing about something from their past and the nurse loudly interrupts and changes the subject.
Mockery	The nurse laughs or makes derogatory comments at the behaviour exhibited by the person.
Disparagement	The nurse makes negative comments to the person such as *You are being really difficult today,* which can lower self-esteem.

Table 3.1: Continued

As can be seen in Table 3.1, there are many things that a nurse might do that may be accepted behaviour in the care culture but can cause harm to the person's sense of themselves.

Activity 3.4 — *Reflection*

Consider when you might have observed any of these MSP behaviours.

Did you recognise that they were a problem?

What could you do, or did you do, about this?

As this is a personal reflection, there is no outline answer at the end of the chapter.

As nurses we are expected to recognise and challenge discriminatory or abusive behaviours such as malignant social psychology (MSP). If we see other nurses practising in this way, we are legally and ethically obliged to raise their awareness of it, and if they do not respond, we need to 'blow the whistle'. The NMC has developed clear guidance on how to raise and escalate concerns (NMC, 2010b). It is important to acknowledge, though, that some nurses may be unaware of their MSP, so the first step is to talk to them about your understanding from your reading of books such as this or Kitwood's.

It has been suggested that it is not the physical or psychological impairment that cause a disability but rather the social and physical environment. While medical and psychological theories support dementia as a disease process, the socio-cultural approach can offer a different view of the experience. Kitwood (1997) offers guidance on how social and environmental elements can also become part of the medical and psychology care given by nurses; see Table 3.2. Although many of these activities, such as play, can be undertaken alone, to support **positive person work** it needs to be an interactive activity.

There are many cultures that do not recognise dementia as a disease, and in Western society it has only more recently been seen as such, mostly since the 1970s (Downs, 2000). The way someone with cognitive impairment such as dementia is viewed will depend on the value base of their culture. Western cultures tend to put a high value on cognitive abilities, and therefore a person with a loss of cognitive ability is devalued. If this impairment is identified as a disease, the person can receive treatment and care, but if it is seen as normal ageing, there is an even greater risk of stigmatisation within our culture and social isolation.

Now that we have examined attitudes, and seen that they derive from culture, we need to look more closely at what we mean by culture.

Culture

A consensual definition of culture found in the literature is that it consists of shared group behaviours and norms, such as traditions, values, beliefs, attitudes, symbols, language, religion and social roles of an ethnic group (Napoles et al., 2010, p390). Kitwood's (1997) more simplified definition is that culture is the patterns of

Positive person work	Examples
Recognition	Greeting the person by name.
Negotiation	Offering the person choices such as when they would like their meal.
Collaboration	Working together on a task such as washing up the dishes.
Play	Doing something just for the pleasure of it, such as dancing.
Timalation	Engaging in a sensual pleasure – for example, massage.
Celebration	Taking the opportunity to express pleasure together, perhaps over the sun shining or seeing a small child play.
Relaxation	Sitting together and listening to music, for example.
Validation	Acknowledging the experience of the person and demonstrating empathy by statements such as, *You appear to be enjoying . . .*
Holding	Holding someone's hand (physical holding) but also giving them space to express strong emotions (psychological holding).
Facilitation	Supporting the person do things they could not do without assistance – maybe playing a musical instrument where you need to hold it in the right position for them.

Table 3.2: Kitwood's (1997) positive person work

behaviour that give meaning to experience and structure for actions for a group. It has been called the 'lens' through which we see the world, and it supports our assumptions about the world. It can be expressed symbolically through language, art and ritual (Draper and McSheery, 2007). Culture, as with attitudes and values, can be experienced explicitly or **implicitly**; we can be consciously aware of our culture, and that of others, or it can influence us at an unconscious level.

There are three main elements to culture: its knowledge or power base; its behavioural norms; and its **ideology** or belief system. Kitwood suggests that dominant cultures are difficult to change, but that the culture of dementia care needs to change in order to provide person-centred care (Kitwood, 1997).

Ideologies underpinning Western culture

Rothman (2000) also suggests that cultures are underpinned by ideologies. These ideologies or world views or, to use the 'lens' analogy again, the direction in which the culture is pointed influence not only how we as nurses interact with those for whom we care but also how we see ourselves. There are three political ideologies that can be recognised in most Western cultures: patriarchy, technology and capitalism. All three of these support a biomedical approach to health (see Chapter 2 for definitions of models of care, including the biomedical approach).

- *Patriarchy* is a system that raises a masculine attitude as more valuable than a feminine one, making health care goal-orientated or task-orientated, focused and audit driven.
- A *technology* or *economy* approach is one where health care and people are viewed in a mechanical way, as systems; it is the ability to function economically that is important, and certain parts should be removed or replaced, if necessary, to achieve this. Economic ideologies do not value those who do not contribute financially to society.
- A *capitalism* approach to health care is one of **commodification**, with health becoming a product (a commodity) that can be bought and sold along with the services of the people who provide it.

So what do these ideologies mean for people with dementia, and their care? Patriarchy could lead to people with dementia having reduced autonomy, and the care given focused on achievement of tasks. The technology ideology would also focus health care on the achievement of tasks, but this would be supported by assistive technology. For example, if a person with dementia has problems with 'wandering' at night, 'cot sides', locked doors, or sedatives may be advocated. Capitalism supports advocacy and choice but only for those who can buy it, so in a purely capitalist society people with dementia who have sufficient funds would be able to buy the type of care they chose, and from whom they chose, but some would have no care provided at all. In the UK, we have the NHS and social services to support and care for people; despite the underlying ideologies, we have a **mixed economy** (private and public funding), which is due to the development of our democratic governmental system.

Western ideologies and humanised care

As we saw in Chapter 2 and will revisit in Chapter 4, a person-centred, holistic approach is advocated for those experiencing dementia. In Western society, the ideologies of patriarchy, technology and capitalism do not support this. Kitwood (1997), Nolan et al. (2004) and Todres et al. (2009) support a humanistic approach. You will probably realise that if our Western culture is underpinned by patriarchy, technology and capitalism, it is going to provide difficult environments in which to provide humanised care.

In the early twenty-first century in the UK we have seen a move towards non-intervention by government, which is a movement away from paternalism towards self-reliance (Forbat, 2008). This promotes self-efficacy and autonomy and is therefore supported by some of the literature related to a person-centred approach. But if autonomy is the focus of care, we risk creating health problems for the families and carers of people with dementia. This is why Nolan et al. (2004) indicated that dementia care should be a triadic (three-way), not a dyadic (two-way) process. By this they mean that care should be negotiated, planned and implemented with the nurse, the person with dementia and their family. The National Dementia Strategy (DH, 2009), produced by the government, incorporates person-centred care, the needs of carers and recognition of the importance of relationships and the environment, something that Forbat (2008) recommends and could be defined as a **whole systems approach**. Despite this, humanised care is still not provided for many of those with dementia (DH, 2010a; CQC, 2011). Although policies have been developed to address research evidence, including people's experiences, they have not changed care for many people with dementia. Why is this? It may be due to the values and attitudes of the nurses implementing care. There has certainly been huge debate in a number of areas – including nursing conferences, nursing press and the national media – due in part to nursing becoming an all-graduate profession and the Care Quality Commission reports about nurses' attitudes and values. These debates have considered issues such as whether nurses lack respect and are 'too posh to wash'. An alternative explanation could be that cultural **hegemony**, the dominant ideology of the culture, does not support a person-centred approach. As indicated by Kitwood (1997), the culture may blind a nurse to malignant social psychology.

The Conservative–Liberal Democrat Alliance in 2011 proposed a new health care bill that is expected to become fully operational in 2013 and lead to the biggest changes to health care in the UK since the introduction of the NHS. The bill states that a new way of commissioning services will put patients at the heart of all they do, providing more patient choice and control. It has created a great deal of discussion and concern as many see this as a movement towards the ideologies of capitalism and technology. Having choices is fine when buying washing machines, but is it appropriate for health care? Not everyone in society is able to make choices on their own.

Cultures within nursing

While the ideologies discussed above underpin Western culture, there are many other smaller micro-cultures or ways of seeing the world that can influence a nurse. We all experience a number of different cultures, including our professional culture, geographical cultures, and religious or ethnic cultures.

The professional culture of nursing has changed in the last few decades. Prior to 1990 nursing was seen primarily as a vocation, which led to nurses being poorly paid and allied with nuns and angels. In the 1980s there was a situation drama on the television entitled *Angels* that followed the lives of a group of student nurses. The title was not explicitly suggesting the nurses were angels – it related to the name of the hospital in which they worked – but there was the implication that nurses were seen as angels. In 1990 Project 2000 was implemented with the aim of getting nurses recognised as autonomous professionals on a par with other health care professionals. Certainly nurses in the twenty-first century do have more autonomy and a greater scope of practice than in the late twentieth century. Many nurses no longer see themselves as 'Florence Nightingale' or a 'comforting angel' but as professionals with a career ladder to climb. Sadly, despite this professionalisation of nursing, malignant social psychology can still be seen to cause problems.

Activity 3.5 — *Reflection*

One in four people in hospital have dementia, and the highest risk factor for having dementia is age. Spend a few moments thinking about what the consequences might be when nurses do not wish to work with older people.

Will they be motivated and compassionate?

Will their care be of the highest quality?

What has influenced your thoughts?

As this is a personal reflection, no outline answer is provided at the end of the chapter.

The professional culture within nursing has changed over time, and the same occurs with other cultures, but for some dominant cultures and religious groups there is a focus on **orthodoxy** and maintaining a strict adherence to certain rules. Nurses are required to support these ethnic and religious needs when giving care. An ethnic group is said to be a group with a *shared heritage, ancestry, religion, language, or common culture* (Napoles et al., 2010, p390).

In the UK the largest ethnic minority group of older people are from South Asia. Many of the older women from this area are unable to read and write in their first language. This could have an impact on whether they gain a diagnosis of dementia. People from ethnic minority groups tested tend to be more likely to be assessed as having a cognitive impairment (Parker and Philp, 2004).

In the US, as with the UK, there is a growing population of older people from immigrant groups with a subsequent increase in those diagnosed with dementia (Napoles et al., 2010). The demographics indicate that there is an urgent need to consider the care required. The literature indicates that the care needs of ethnic groups are different from those of the non-latino-white majority, but the studies appear to suggest that care is not being culturally tailored (Napoles et al., 2010). The Centre for Cultural Diversity in Aging (2011), with particular reference to dementia care, identified that the most important aspect of care to ensure it is culturally sensitive is language and communication.

All of the models of care that were described in Chapter 2 and that will be further explored in Chapter 7 address the concern for culturally sensitive care as they are individualistic, assessing the holistic care needs of the person and the person in relation to their families and social groups. They support the need for communication that demonstrates respect for the person and maintains their dignity. As part of this it is important, as far as is possible, to provide information and care in the person's first language so that they have the best opportunity not only to understand but also to interact with their caregiver.

People with dementia will increasingly have difficulty with verbal communication. If people have language differences, assessing how their dementia is affecting their ability to communicate is challenging (Parker and Philp, 2004). It is well documented that older people in black and ethnic minority groups are more likely to be assessed on dementia screening tools as having a cognitive impairment than white British (Parker and Philp, 2004). One of the reasons offered for this is that the measures are culturally biased. Consider the case study of Aastha Patel and how assessing any cognitive impairment may be difficult.

Case study: Aastha Patel

Aastha, whose name means faith, arrived in the UK when she was a young woman to marry a man whom her parents had chosen for her. She had been living in a rural area of the Indian subcontinent and only had a few words of English when she arrived; her first language was Gujarati. Aastha is a Hindu and, as indicated by her name, she has been a woman of faith throughout her life. She has been happily married for 40 years, and her children have grown up and left home. Aastha had taken the opportunities provided in her local community to learn to speak, read and write English, although when her family were at home together they spoke Gujarati. She encouraged her children and grandchildren to learn and be mindful of their god, to recognise their oneness with nature and the power of chanting. Aastha chooses to wear the traditional sari, but her children and husband wear more Western-style clothing. Aastha and her husband are vegetarian, as are most Hindus.

Aastha's first language is Gujarati; at times of distress or if she had dementia, it is likely she would revert to using her primary language. There is also the likelihood, given Aastha's home in her childhood, that she would not have received a Western-style education. These two factors, language and education, are suggested as the main reasons for underperformance of ethnic groups on cognitive impairment scales.

Common test items when screening for dementia involve:

- orientation to time;
- orientation to place;
- attention/concentration;
- memory for previously learnt information;
- memory for new information;
- language;
- visuospatial skills.
  (Parker and Philp, 2004)

Activity 3.6   *Critical thinking*

Consider how Aastha might answer the questions or undertake the activities below.

Questions
- What is the date?
- Where do you live?
- When was the Second World War?
- What is your date of birth?

continued . . .

Activities
- Spell a word backwards.
- Do some numerical additions.
- Undertake an action such as putting one book on top of another.
- Complete a half-drawn shape.
  (Parker and Philp, 2004)

An outline answer is given at the end of the chapter.

All of the common test items may have specific problems for people like Aestha who come from a minority ethnic group, but a number of tests have been translated into a variety of languages. An example is the mini mental state examination (MMSE), which is one of the mostly commonly used tools for assessing dementia (Parker and Philp, 2004). This tool, though, has a high false positive rate associated with educational ability and language. Other tools, such as the clock drawing test and the time and change tests, have been found to be more reliable and acceptable to older people from ethnic minorities (Parker and Philp, 2004). Assessment is discussed in more detail in Chapter 5.

Culture and carers

It is emphasised throughout this book that nurses need to take into consideration the primary caregiver for the person with dementia; this is frequently the spouse or another family member. A person's culture will have a big impact on how their family is organised and the behavioural norms within it. Some of the care-giving norms of different cultural groups are set out below.

- *African-American caregivers*: This group values role over cognitive ability, so if the person with dementia can still fulfil a role, they remain a valuable member of the family and are not seen as in need of care. This reduces the stress or burden felt by the caregiver and also reduces their support seeking (Gallagher-Thompson et al., 2003).
- *Hispanic/Latino American caregivers*: For this group dementia is stigmatised, as it is seen as mental disorder or normal ageing. They have a complex combined belief system related to health and illness that leads to high levels of carer stress and burden (Gallagher-Thompson et al., 2003).
- *Chinese American*: This group views dementia as either part of normal ageing or as mental disorder, which leads to stigmatisation and a lack of help-seeking behaviour (Downs, 2000).

Despite these suggested cultural stereotypes, there is great variation within cultures in caring for a person with dementia.

Activity 3.7   *Reflection*

Take a few minutes to think about your family.

- Who do you feel belongs to your family? Are they all biologically related?
- Do you have a group outside your biological relations that you call family, such as a church family?
- What behavioural norms and values do you share?
- Think about how your family values might affect how you view other families.

If you know someone who has a diagnosis of dementia, consider the following questions related them – if not, think what might happen.

- How do others behave towards them?
- Do they retain their status within the family?

As this is a personal reflection, there is no outline answer at the end of the chapter.

Providing culturally sensitive care is an essential part of the nurse's role in caring for people with dementia (Boise, 2008). To give this type of care, we, as nurses, need to consider the person and their family's views of dementia. These are some questions you could use to guide your assessment of their care needs.

- What do they think dementia is?
- Do they think it is a normal part of ageing?
- Do they feel it is important that others do not know about the condition?
- What are the strengths and abilities of the person with dementia?
- What support do they have and need?
- How do they think dementia progresses? What is its trajectory?

Many cultures recognise dementia either as part of normal ageing or as a mental disorder, and this will affect how they respond to it. As was suggested by Gallagher-Thompson et al. (2003) and Downs (2000), viewing dementia as a normal part of ageing may lead to a lack of seeking help; likewise viewing dementia as a mental disorder could lead to stigmatisation. It may also be that accepting cognitive impairment as normal ageing facilitates acceptance and a reduced feeling of burden for the family. It is therefore important that nurses approach the person and their family with sensitivity.

The key issues in overcoming cultural barriers in dementia care are language, low education, cultural beliefs about dementia, knowledge and attitudes of carers/family (Alagiakrishnan, 2008). As nurses we need to develop skills to reduce or ameliorate these barriers. Some ways in which you could do this are:

- identifying the primary language of the person, accessing interpreters and seeking translated literature;
- talking to the person and their family about their beliefs, understandings and rituals.
- introducing them to others in similar situations so that they can share knowledge, under- standing and support.

A person's culture provides behavioural norms, support through recognised relationships and an understanding about the world. Another significant element of a person's culture is that it can provide meaning for their lives – their spirituality.

Spirituality

In the twentieth century there was little recognition given to spirituality in health care in the UK, perhaps as a response to the fervent evangelism of the Victorian Christians or the growth in our multi-cultural society. Spirituality and religious activities have, though, been closely linked to health and well-being throughout history, with health care in medieval Britain provided in monasteries and convents. The old psychiatric hospitals, mostly now closed, had their beautiful chapels, and we can find small places of worship or meditation in most UK hospitals today. It is important to recognise that historically, spirituality was closely linked to particular religions, whereas we now have a broader definition of spirituality.

Verity and Lee (2011) suggest that the spirit is the 'spark of life' in people. It is this spark of life that demonstrates their well-being; a common saying when someone is depressed or particularly unwell is that the 'sparkle' or 'light' has gone out of their eyes. This is something that has also been suggested for people who experience dementia; the spark of life – the small light that was the person – appears diminished. In this situation the spirit of the person is identified as having left the body. This part of the chapter, though, is going to challenge this view of the person with dementia.

Spirituality is defined as *That which lies at the core of each person's being, an essential dimension which brings meaning to life* (MacKinlay, 2001, p52). As such, we can see its importance in dementia care nursing. As memory and confusion increase, a sense of meaning for life can bring hope and facilitate coping strategies. MacKinlay (2011), in her model of spirituality adapted for those with dementia, identifies that transcending loss, finding hope and intimacy with God or in relationship with others are significant features that interact with a sense of meaning for the person. The basis of MacKinlay's (2011) model is that spirituality is mediated through religion, relationships, environment and arts. Read the case study of Olivia in the box to gain an insight into her spirituality, and use Activity 3.8 to explore what this means to her.

Case study: Olivia Olsen

Olivia is 69 and she has a diagnosis of Alzheimer's dementia. Her husband was a member of the clergy, and she attended Christian church services on Sundays to support her husband, even when their children were young. Since his death she has gradually become more forgetful and confused. Olivia now struggles to dress herself appropriately and is unable to find her own way to the church for services. She remembers her husband is dead but gets confused about when she last saw her children and how old they are; when prompted, she does remember their names. On arrival at the church for a service she is frequently tearful and confused.

As soon as the music starts, Olivia is reawakened. She joins in with the singing of hymns, remembering all the words. She joins in with prayers, her face brightens and she experiences her relationship with God. At the end of the service she enjoys interacting with the other churchgoers and remains refreshed for a while.

Activity 3.8 — *Critical thinking*

What is spirituality for Olivia?

How does Olivia gain meaning in her life?

How does her spirituality support her sense of well being?

An outline answer is provided at the end of the chapter.

Spirituality can be seen to be important for Olivia's sense of well-being, but another element of her spirituality is the ritual involved. Ritual can facilitate a response and interaction with a person's spirituality or engagement with the meaning of life for them.

Religion is one element of spirituality in MacKinlay's model (2011). A useful definition of religion is that it is a system of faith and worship that usually involves one or more greater being/s – god/s who have control and deserve worship and obedience. Most organised religion has its set rituals, and if we consider the case study of Olivia, we can see how involvement in religious rituals has facilitated access to memories and a sense of well-being for her.

Rituals, though, do not have to be religious. They can involve everyday activities such as preparation for bed or eating a meal. Most rituals use symbols. For Olivia, the symbols used were the place – the church and the ornamentation such as religious icons – but probably the most influential for her was the music, the chanting of liturgy (music and song have a huge impact on memory; see Chapter 7) and the types of interactions engaged in. Many activities have ritualistic elements; the case study of Gareth will allow you to explore this idea a little more.

Case study: Gareth Collier

Gareth was a coal miner for 40 years and retired at 58 on health grounds; his breathing had become progressively difficult. Gareth now also has a diagnosis of dementia. He is a proud man and very proud of his mining ancestry; in his youth he was considered the strongest and fittest young man in the local villages. Despite many of his peers attending chapel he could not accept an all-powerful god and considered himself an atheist.

Throughout his life he has fished as a hobby, and although he is now escorted when he goes fishing, he appears to gain a sense of meaning for himself and the world by undertaking this activity. Despite failing memory and confusion, when his son comes to take him fishing he is able to find and collect all his fishing gear. They walk to the river without his son prompting him which way to go, and he is able to set up his rod, bait his line and flick the rod to get the 'hook, line and sinker' in the best fishing spot. When Gareth sits down with his rod, he can peacefully watch the river with a look of contentment on his face and tell his son fluent stories of previous fishing episodes in great detail.

Activity 3.9   *Critical thinking*

Read the case study of Gareth Collier.

Do you think fishing is a spiritual activity for him?

Is there any ritualistic behaviour involved?

What symbols are used in fishing? What impact do they appear to have on Gareth's experience of dementia?

An outline answer is provided at the end of this chapter.

It can be seen in the case study of Gareth that spirituality for him is more to do with his ability to find comfort, self-acceptance and a sense of place where he can be who he is. This was the same for Olivia: her spirituality, expressed through the church service, provides meaning in her life, self-acceptance, a sense of belonging and place, and she is able to be Olivia, an embodied and significant person. The sense of being an embodied and significant person is important to gain a sense of well-being for all of us.

Spirituality links with Erikson's virtues, Kitwood's and Maslow's needs and Nolan et al.'s senses, as described in Chapter 2. This is particularly the case for Nolan et al.'s need for a sense of significance, Erikson's achievement of the virtue of wisdom, Kitwood's need for comfort and Maslow's achievement of self-actualisation.

Through this discussion you should be able to recognise how important it is that you address the person's spiritual needs when providing nursing care. To do this requires an individualistic, person-centred, humanised approach to care, as each person will have different ways of gaining and expressing spirituality, as can be seen in the case studies. An assessment style that facilitates this is story telling; the person, perhaps helped by their family, shares their life story with you.

The understanding gained from this short exploration of spirituality can be applied to your nursing interactions to increase spirituality and develop a sense of well-being for those with dementia in some very practical ways. For example, rituals are important for people, especially those with reduced memory capacity and confusion, as was seen in the case studies of Olivia and Gareth. As a nurse you could check what rituals the person or their family usually use in a given situation such as bathing or eating. The Alzheimer's Society leaflet 'This is me' is a useful tool to gain this information. You could then use the same ritual in your care of them, so they understand what is happening and can be more independent.

Spirituality encompasses religion, relationships, environment and art (MacKinlay 2011), and as a nurse you need to be mindful of these.

- How can you facilitate attendance at religious or significant social events?
- Does the environment in which someone is living enhance their sense of meaning and self?
- Does the person have the opportunity for self-expression through art, such as dancing, singing and painting?

The way in which you achieve these to provide spiritual care will depend on the individuals involved, but these are key areas for you to consider.

Chapter summary

The key point that can be drawn from this chapter is the need to treat people with respect as embodied and significant people who may have different cultures and belief systems from you. You, as a nurse, should not make general assumptions but check with the individual and their family about their attitudes, values and beliefs and, where possible, address these. Many people in our society have different ethnic cultures, which will have an influence on how well they perform using certain assessment tools. When assessing or caring you need to ensure you use culturally sensitive approaches. Spirituality encompasses religion, relationships, environment and art (MacKinlay, 2011). To address spiritual needs can increase the person's self-acceptance, comfort and sense of well-being.

Activities: brief outline answers

Activity 3.1: Critical thinking (page 43)

Martin and Sarah appear to have developed the attitude that to achieve things effort is needed. They have both received and given love/care, so this is probably important to them.

Martin may also have developed a risk-averse attitude given his experience with his brother, and Sarah may have developed an attitude that personal expression, if necessary against social norms, is important.

Martin's attitude towards risk may encourage him to restrict choices and autonomy for the people he works with to keep them safe, while Sarah may put less effort into reducing risk and more into ensuring empowerment and autonomy.

Both attitudes could be useful or a problem for the people they care for. When caring for a person with dementia Sarah may not restrict behaviours that could cause harm to the person, whereas Martin may reduce their quality of life and esteem by putting in place too many restrictions. If Martin and Sarah are aware of their own and each other's value base and attitudes, they could work together to ensure safety and empowerment.

Activity 3.3: Critical thinking (page 45)

The unit nurse has not spoken to Bruno, sought his consent or asked for any information from him. This could be based on the assumption that Bruno is unable to give consent or provide the nurse with the information they need.

This could be based on a negative stereotype that Bruno is unable to understand what is happening and lacks competence to make decisions for himself. It could also be based on information provided by his escort from the nursing home.

This is discriminatory behaviour, probably based on negative stereotyping. The *Essence of care* document (DH, 2010d) gives clear guidance on effective communication, and the Mental Capacity Act (DH, 2005/2007) clearly states that nurses should always assume people are competent to make decisions (explored in more detail in Chapter 8), unless an assessment of incompetence has been established for this particular occasion. The nurse has also not shown respect for Bruno and denied him dignity in this situation.

Activity 3.6: Critical thinking (pages 52–3)

What is the date?

This requires a familiarity with Western calendars that might not have been part of Astha's early experience or particularly necessary in her current everyday life. It is important to point out that some people who have been immersed in Western culture also struggle with this, especially if they have spent some time in the US as the UK date is arranged day/month/year, but in the US it is arrange month/day/year.

Where do you live?

This requires an understanding of how addresses are organised. A person immersed in the UK culture would probably respond to this without thinking, but a person who is unsure of what is expected may respond by naming the people they live with.

When was the Second World War? What is your date of birth?

Many people in the world do not have a date of birth as their birth was not recorded. They would therefore not be able to answer this question. There might be similar problems to the other date question at the beginning of this activity. As Aastha would have been a small child living in rural India at the time of the Second World War, it may not be part of her memory and it may not have been something of the highest priority for her family to talk to her about as she grew up.

Spell a word backwards or do some numerical additions

If Aastha is anxious or has some limited cognitive impairment due to a minor infection or due to dementia, she may not be able to undertake this task due to her lack of Western education and English not being her first language.

Undertake an action such as putting one book on top of another.

This task may create problems for Aastha in a similar way to others. She may not understand the request, and, even if she does, it may not make sense in terms of real-world activity. She may be able to perform many complex tasks that she may encounter in everyday experience but not a simple task in this setting because she does not understand what is expected.

Complete a half-drawn shape

To complete a half-drawn shape assumes the person knows what the complete shape would look like, and many shapes that are familiar to us may not be to a person who did not experience a Western education.

Activity 3.8: Critical thinking (page 56)

Spirituality for Olivia involves a belief system that acknowledges and responds to a monotheist religion. Through this she gains an understanding that all life is under submission to God, an all-powerful being, to whom she should offer worship and interact with through prayer. Considering MacKinlay's model (2011), Olivia's spirituality or sense of meaning is derived through her relationship with God, her engagement with God's creation (nature, sea, mountains etc.), religious ritual (prayer, worship, liturgy) and the arts (music, dance etc.). Spirituality supports Olivia's sense of well-being by allowing her to recognise that her life and others, however problematic, have meaning and she has worth. She can achieve a sense of peace and comfort through engagement in religious rituals, relationships and the arts, which facilitate recall of activities, events and emotions.

Activity 3.9: Critical thinking (page 57)

For some, like Gareth, fishing could be seen as engagement with spirituality. Fishing provides a sense of well-being for him and enables him to be more in touch with who he is; it could therefore be said to provide some meaning for his life. While fishing he engages with his environment and is able to manage his close relationship with his son. Fishing is, for some, recognised as an art.

There were a number of rituals in which Gareth took part in during his fishing trip. There was the ritual of organising his gear, the ritual of setting up his rod, and the ritual of sitting and waiting. The reminiscing with his son may also be considered ritualistic.

Many symbols can be found in this activity: the symbols of clothing, the equipment, the river and maybe even his son. All the rituals, symbols and spiritual engagement have facilitated a sense of well-being and peace for Gareth; it has also improved his recall and communication skills.

Further reading

Boise, L (2008) Ethnicity and the experience of dementia, in Downs, M and Bower, B (eds) *Excellence in dementia care: research into practice.* Maidenhead: McGraw Hill Open University Press: 52–70.

Linda Boise offers a clear, concise overview of the research and understanding of how culture and ethnicity impact on help-seeking behaviours, the barriers people face and how research in this area can be applied to practice.

Kitwood, T (1997) *Dementia reconsidered: the person comes first.* Maidenhead: Open University Press.

This book has been reprinted many times, and it is seen as a core text for exploring a person-centred approach to dementia care.

Mackinlay, E (2011) Creative processes to bring out expressions of spirituality: working with people who have dementia, in Lee, H and Adams, T (eds) *Creative approaches in dementia care.* Basingstoke: Palgrave: 212–29.

Elizabeth Mackinlay has researched and written in the area of spirituality for a number of years, and in this chapter she gives an overview of her research, the model she developed and its application in practice.

Useful websites

http://alzheimers.org.uk/site/scripts/download_info.php?fileID=454

The *Out of the shadows* report on the experience of stigma by those with dementia has been developed by the Alzheimer's Society.

www.dementiacentre.com

The Dementia Centre offers information and support for people with dementia, their carers, family and health care professionals.

www.nmc-uk.org/Documents/Guidance/Guidance-for-the-care-of-older-people.pdf

Although the NMC guidance for the care of older people does not directly refer to dementia, it gives clear guidance on how to support anti-discriminatory practice and the elements of spirituality raised in this chapter.

Chapter 4
The person

```
···················································································
:  ·  ·  ·          NMC Standards for Pre-registration Nursing Education  :
:                                                                         :
```

This chapter will address issues within all four domains of the pre-registration nursing competencies but most significantly the following:

Domain 1: Professional values

4. All nurses must work in partnership with service users, carers, families, groups, communities and organisations. They must manage risk, and promote health and wellbeing while aiming to empower choices that promote self-care and safety.

Domain 3: Nursing practice and decision-making

4. All nurses must ascertain and respond to the physical, social and psychological needs of people, groups and communities. They must then plan, deliver and evaluate safe, competent, person-centred care in partnership with them, paying special attention to changing health needs during different life stages, including progressive illness and death, loss and bereavement.

```
···················································································
:  ·  ·  ·  ·                            NMC Essential Skills Clusters  :
:                                                                         :
```

This chapter will support the following ESCs:

Cluster: Care, compassion and communication

2. People can trust the newly registered graduate nurse to engage in person centred care empowering people to make choices about how their needs are met when they are unable to meet them for themselves.

Cluster: Organisational aspects of care

10. People can trust the newly registered graduate nurse to deliver nursing interventions and evaluate their effectiveness against the agreed assessment and care plan.

By entry to the register:

vi. Provides safe and effective care in partnership with people and their carers within the context of people's ages, conditions and developmental stages.

> ## Chapter aims
>
> On completion of this chapter you should have developed an understanding of:
>
> - person and personhood;
> - ageing through the lifespan;
> - recognition of the importance of family and carer in personhood and humanisation.

Introduction

Terry Pratchett, a renowned author, said, *It seems that when you have cancer you are a brave battler against the disease, but when you have Alzheimer's you are an old fart. That's how people see you. It makes you feel quite alone* (Pratchett, 2008). In October 2011 the *Daily Mail* discussed the Care Quality Commission's report on the provision of nutrition and dignity in the NHS (CQC, 2011), which *found one in five NHS hospitals are providing care so neglectful that it is breaking the law* (*Daily Mail*, 2011). Both of these statements are shocking, and it is saddening that people in our affluent society are having these experiences. This chapter focuses on a person-centred approach – a respectful and humanised approach that will facilitate your understanding of the person with dementia. It will consider what it means to be a 'person' and discuss personhood through psychological theory related to lifespan development.

The person

As nurses, it may be *obvious to us that people are different and unique; common sense offers us a number of ways of differentiating: culture, gender, temperament, social class, lifestyle, outlook, beliefs, values commitments, tastes, interests – and so on* (Kitwood, 1997, p15). Consider the case study of Nathan and Jordan; they were brought up in the same culture, are the same gender, the same social class and probably have the same values. If they needed nursing care for dementia, would it be appropriate to offer them the same care?

> ### Case study: Nathan and Jordan Cohen
>
> *Nathan and Jordan are brothers, and there is only a year between them in age. Nathan, the older brother, is dark haired and tall, whereas Jordan is blonde and small, but both have a thick head of curly hair. Both brothers are intelligent and made great achievements at school and university. Nathan was always in charge when the brothers did anything together, and Jordan always hung back in his brother's shadow, not wishing to be on display. Nathan enjoys football and rugby, but Jordan prefers computer games and chess. Nathan always seems full of energy while Jordan is quite content to sit and watch his brother's antics. They both have a good understanding of their abilities and appear self-confident and happy with who they are.*

Nathan and Jordan are different people despite having many things in common, so Nathan might be able to express himself in social activities and groups, but this might be something that would make Jordan uncomfortable. If Nathan's social contact was restricted, he might become low in mood and frustrated.

Activity 4.1   *Reflection*

Spend a few minutes thinking about what makes you a person.

When you meet someone for the first time what information do you give about yourself or ask of them?

Perhaps you give your name. Do you include your family name? Do you offer your usual occupation? Your marital status? Where you live? Your interests?

Are these the things that make you distinct from everyone else?

Is there something else that makes you unique? Or do you think that there are groups or types of people?

As this is a personal reflection, there is no outline answer at the end of the chapter.

What does it mean to be a person?

Rewston and Moniz-Cook (2008) state that recognising and understanding psychological approaches can enhance dementia care. Psychology, which seeks to study people and the way they think, feel and interact with others, offers us a variety of perspectives to understand what it is to be a person. The theoretical work related to the person is normally considered under the heading of personality, within which psychologists seek to determine individual differences, types and influencing factors (Brinich and Shelley, 2002). Personality can be defined as the features of a person that are fairly stable and enduring, which allow them to be compared to others but at the same time make them unique (Barker, 2007).

Uniqueness and individuality have an important philosophical position in Western cultures, but, as with other values and beliefs, they have been adopted as our culture has developed. See Chapter 3 for a further exploration of culture. It is only in the last couple of hundred years that viewing people as individuals has been the accepted norm in our culture. Our Western conception of people as individuals developed during the Victorian romanticism and the modernism of the late twentieth century, although it does have some earlier roots (Brinich and Shelley, 2002). The ideology of individualism is firmly engrained in Western ways of thinking. While this chapter, immersed in the pervading culture, focuses on the uniqueness of individuals, it also recognises that people are not isolated in a vacuum; all people are in relationship with others. This chapter therefore takes the journey of exploring the individual and moves on to consider people in relationships.

Personality and lifespan development

The five main perspectives in psychology that guide our exploration of the person are recognised as: biological, behavioural, cognitive, psychodynamic and humanistic (Barker, 2007). All of these perspectives are useful in guiding nurses' understanding of the person and their care of people with dementia. They also offer an understanding of the lifespan development of the person. The biological and psychodynamic theories articulate distinct stages of development and change throughout the lifespan, whereas behavioural and humanistic approaches offer an understanding that applies to all ages. The cognitive approach offers a childhood developmental theory, but most of the changes in later life appear to be related to physiological (biological) changes.

Biological psychology

The biological psychologists identify biological differences when establishing the uniqueness of individuals, and they see developmental and maturational changes of the nervous and endocrine systems as influential in both behaviour and emotions. The nervous system develops rapidly in childhood, but it continues to adapt and change in adulthood. During babyhood and infancy (0–2 years) the brain grows to 70 per cent of its adult size and by early childhood (2–6 years) it reaches 90 per cent of its adult size. Although in middle childhood (6–12 years) **neuronal plasticity** declines, in adolescence **synaptic growth** and **myelinisation** are still very active (Berk, 2008) – see the theory summary box for an explanation of these terms. Biological development is usually divided into stages: pre-birth, infancy, early childhood, middle childhood, adolescence, young adulthood, middle adulthood, late adulthood (late adulthood has also been divided into three stages since the increase in life expectancy). In each of these stages significant physical/biological changes can be seen.

Theory summary: biological terms

neurone	another name for a nerve cell.
neuronal	pertaining to a nerve cell.
neuronal plasticity or *neuroplasticity*	the nerve's potential to adapt to changes or injury that can be chemical or structural:

- structurally, the neurone can grow more dendrites (projections from the main cell body) to form new synapses or dendrites can retract or shrivel and reduce synapses.
- chemically, nerves can become more sensitive to certain chemicals, increase or decrease production of chemicals.

synapse	where one neurone meets another, they do not grow together; to communicate, neurotransmitters are released from one neurone and passed to the next across a small gap; this gap is what is known as a synapse.
synaptic pruning	the reduction of synapses.

myelinisation	the process of attaching a myelin coat (made of cholesterol) to the neurone. Myelin sheaths (coats) facilitate increased speed of neurones and offer them protection.

Activity 4.2 — Critical thinking

You are caring for an adolescent aged 13. What might you need to take into consideration in relation to this stage of the lifespan?

An outline answer can be found at the end of the chapter.

Despite the reduction in neural plasticity in middle childhood, the body continues to develop until the person is about 20 years old, i.e. into young adulthood. At this point some decline in a number of areas can be seen. There is a decline in sensations such as touch and systems such as respiration, cardiovascular and immunity, but the person is usually at their peak for coordination and strength. In their thirties and forties the person can expect reduced performance in their sight and hearing and their hair may start to become grey. In the forties to sixties there is a reduction in lean body mass (muscle and bone) (Berk, 2008). While this paints a rather negative picture of ageing, it is not all bad news: neuronal plasticity continues facilitating learning and adaptation, hence the 'wisdom of age'.

Neuronal plasticity can offer us an understanding of why someone may have extensive brain cell death due to insufficient blood supply, **neural fibrillary tangles**, **plaques** or Lewy bodies and not demonstrate any of the symptoms associated with dementia. A lot of research has been conducted in this area, leading to treatment of dementia with certain drugs; see Chapter 7.

Hans J Eysenck (1916–1997) proposed that personality was biologically based, and he established three dimensions, or super traits, of personality: introversion–extroversion, neuroticism and psychoticism.

- Introversion – shy and retiring.
- Extroversion – outgoing and assertive.
- Neuroticism – anxious and emotionally unstable.
- Psychoticism – cold and antisocial.

Introversion–extroversion is said to be a **continuum**, so a person may be at one end and be extremely introverted or at the other end and be extremely extroverted or somewhere in-between. Neuroticism or emotionally unstable is one end of a continuum, and emotionally stable is at the other end. Likewise, psychoticism or anti-social is one end of a continuum, and sociability is at the other. Where the person is on these continuums is said to be stable over time and leads to certain traits that facilitate specific responses. For example, if a person is introverted and stable (lacks neuroticism), they may have these traits: calm, even tempered, reliable, controlled, peaceful, thoughtful and careful (Burger, 2011). Although these traits are said to remain throughout the lifespan, evidence suggests that both men and women become more introverted with age and that both neuroticism and psychoticism reduce with age, but on the whole there is little change (Stuart-Hamilton, 2000).

There has been a lot of research in the area of trait theories, and while Eysenck continued to identity his super traits as the most significant, there is evidence to support the existence of five traits, known as the 'big five'. They are:

- extroversion;
- agreeableness;
- conscientiousness;
- emotional stability;
- intellect/openness to experience.

Each of these traits can be seen to be poles, with desirable elements at one end and undesirable elements at the other. For extroversion we can find assertiveness versus passivity, whereas for agreeableness we could have kind and warm at one end and hostile and cold at the other. For conscientiousness we could find tidy at one end and unreliable at the other, and for emotional stability we could have calm versus moody, and with intellect we could have imaginative versus shallow (Gross, 2001).

Activity 4.3   *Reflection*

Take a few minutes and think about your characteristics.

Do you consider yourself extroverted or introverted?

Were you like this as a child?

Have your characteristics changed?

Talk to your parents or older people in your nursing group. Have their characteristics changed over time?

As this is a personal reflection, there is no outline answer at the end of the chapter.

Behavioural psychology

Behavioural psychologists focus on what can be observed and the environment in which the observed behaviour occurs. They suggest that people learn to be the person they are through their interaction with their environment. They do not offer a staged theory of development; they suggest that people are born with the ability and motivation to learn, which occurs through a number of processes. These processes have a high correlation with the neural plasticity explored by the biological psychologists (Kolb and Whishaw, 2006). According to their theories, learning continues throughout an animal's (including a person's) life unless there is a biological reason against it. More primitive animals only learn by the lower level processes, whereas higher functioning animals learn at all levels. The processes of learning developed by the behaviourists are:

- *habituation* – the simplest process, where an organism gets used to a **stimulus** (habituates to it);
- *classical conditioning* – learning by association, so when one stimulus gains a certain **response**, another stimulus presented at the same time over a sustained period will eventually produce the response without the original stimulus;
- *operant conditioning* – learning occurs at this level when a voluntary behaviour is rewarded.

While the theories of classical and operant conditioning have been influential and useful in understanding and changing behaviour, some researchers felt there was more occurring in the individual than a response to a certain environment: a stimulus. They went on to develop the cognitive theories of the person.

Bandura's social learning theory or social cognitive theory indicates that people learn through thinking about things (thought processes) as well as through instinctual (biological prepared) learning processes. As with the early behaviourists, Bandura does not provide a staged development, and he accepts that people learn throughout their lifespan. He states that people learn from the processes already identified but also **vicariously** through observing others. A key element of this learning is through **role models**. This can easily be seen in nurse education where student nurses are given a mentor as a role model to develop their clinical practice.

Using Bandura's social learning theory, we can see that people develop their personality throughout their lifespan by interacting with their environment. This theoretical standpoint offers **self-efficacy** as a key element in personality development and maintenance. Self-efficacy refers to the power or control a person feels they have over their experience and environment. If the person believes they can achieve something, they will try to do it. If a person has high self-efficacy, therefore, they will attempt to undertake things that a person with low self-efficacy will not.

Case study: Elsie Hardwicke

Elsie worked as a nanny until she married her husband and then spent her time caring for her children and husband. She felt fulfilled in her role as she gained pleasure from caring for others, but she has low self-efficacy and relies on her husband to make the decisions and manage their budget. She has recently been diagnosed with Alzheimer's dementia.

Activity 4.4   *Critical thinking*

Given what you know about self-efficacy and Elsie, how do you think Elsie might respond to her diagnosis? What might be your aim in caring for her?

An outline answer is given at the end of the chapter.

Bandura's social learning theory was later renamed social cognitive theory because of its focus on internal processes (cognitive) as well as the environment (social). Other cognitive theorists also accept these two components as being important in the development and maintenance of the personality, but they put more emphasis on internal processes (mental/cognitive).

Cognitive psychology

Cognitive psychologists offer us, as nurses, a staged developmental theory (Piaget's developmental theory) as well as theories related to how people think. Thinking is said to be an essential element of being and recognising oneself as a person, as declared by René Descartes, an influential philosopher: *I think, therefore I am.*

The cognitive developmental theory of Jean Piaget (1896–1980) states that children think in a qualitatively different way from adults. His developmental theory is maturational: children progress naturally through the stages as long as there are no impediments such as mental or physical health problems or a restricted environment.

Piaget's theory is based on **schema theory**, a theory that memory (mental or physical) is stored in packets or groups. This includes how a person views themselves; they have a self-schema or self-concept. Children and adults develop these schemas by processes of **assimilation** and **accommodation**. Assimilation occurs when a person gains new information and adapts an already held schema about a concept, whereas accommodation occurs when a person gains new information, finds it cannot be included in an existing schema, and therefore changes the existing schema or makes a new one.

Cognitive psychologists frequently separate out the different elements of cognition in order to study them. Significant areas are intelligence, memory and problem solving, and each of these can be seen to be parts or **constructs** of the personality.

For all three areas there are changes throughout the lifespan. It is difficult to determine whether the changes are beneficial or a problem, but they will change how the person is viewed and how they view themselves. As people age they tend to depend on **intuitive** problem solving rather than **deductive reasoning**, while for young people it is vice versa. In some circumstances the reliance on experience and intuition can improve problem solving, but for some the more methodical approach of deductive reasoning is needed. While there is a decline in **fluid intelligence** with age, older adults can compensate using their **crystallised intelligence**. Fluid intelligence is physiologically dependent and involves activities such as perceptual speed and visual organisation. Crystallised intelligence is more experientially dependent and includes abilities such as knowledge for general information and verbal comprehension. Over the age of 85 there is a general decline in functioning in intelligence tests (Lefrancois, 1999).

The ability to remember things as people get older is mostly unchanged. Young children are accumulating memory and understanding as the brain adapts and grows. It is recognised that for those between 60 and 80 there is a decrease in **short-term memory** from nine to seven digits but relative stability in **non-declarative memory** – memory for how to do something like tie your shoes – and **semantic memory** – understanding. **Episodic memory** is generally recognised to be a problem for those over 70 in particular (Lefrancois, 1999). This would not appear to be surprising, given that the older the person is the more episodes they need to remember, many of which will be very similar.

For cognitive psychologists, personality can be seen to have a number of parts that come together as a self-schema or self-concept, and a person can play different roles and be perceived to be a different person in different situations.

Psychodynamic psychology

The psychodynamic approach, founded by Sigmund Freud (1896–1939), offers an understanding of the **dynamic** nature of the personality and how a child develops through their interaction with their environment into the mature adult. Freud indicated that, when born, a baby's personality consists purely of innate drives; the baby is a bundle of **id**. Through the psychosexual stages of oral, anal, phallic, latency and genital the child develops a **superego**, a conscience that incorporates the social rules and norms. These two opposing, hence dynamic, parts of the personality are balanced by the **ego**. The ego seeks to achieve the wants, needs and desires of the id within the social parameters of the superego.

Over- or under-stimulation at any of the psychosexual stages will promote certain personality traits. For example, over- or under-stimulation in the anal stage can lead to an anally retentive or anally expulsive personality. An anally expulsive person is untidy and disorganised whereas an anally retentive person is obsessively tidy and organised. Freud also identified the concept of **mental defence mechanisms**, which have an impact on the behaviour of the person, causing people to believe that their personality has changed. These are coping strategies that a person may use when in a crisis and can be useful in the short term (Barker, 2007). Some examples are:

- denial – denying something, such as diagnosis of dementia, has happened;
- projection – suggesting that someone else has the negative feeling, thought, behaviour that they themselves have; for example, a person experiences memory problems but says it is their partner's poor memory that is the problem;
- displacement – transferring a feeling away from the cause on to to something or someone else. For example, a person is angry because they cannot get the support they need from the doctor so they complain about their children's behaviour;
- rationalisation – finding a rational explanation for irrational behaviour. For example, a person walks around a car park four times looking into the cars; when asked if anything is wrong, they reply that they are just thinking about what sort of new car to buy.

Since the early work of Freud there have been a number of theorists who have developed his theory.

Erik Erikson (1902–1994), a student of Freud, developed the psychodynamic theory to incorporate a more social approach; his theory was labelled the psychosocial theory of development. In outline, people continue to develop their ego, their personality, throughout the lifespan through eight crises or stages of change. In each stage an ego strength or virtue is achieved – see Table 4.1 (and also Chapter 2).

Each element of the crisis needs balancing to achieve the virtue or ego strength and to move on to the next stage and maintain a healthy ego. If a crisis is not balanced at the chronological age stated, the person can move on and revisit the crisis at a later stage, but this will cause psychosocial problems for them. For Erikson, it is important that the person maintains and develops their role in society to achieve a sense of well-being.

Stage	Crisis	Virtue/ego strength
1. 0–18 months	Trust versus Mis-trust	Hope
2. 18 months–3 years	Autonomy versus shame	Will
3. 3–6 years	Initiative versus guilt	Purpose
4. 6–puberty	Industry versus inferiority	Skill
5. Adolescence	Identity versus identity confusion	Fidelity
6. Young adulthood	Intimacy versus isolation	Love
7. Middle adulthood	Generativity versus stagnation	Care
8. Older adulthood	Ego integrity versus despair	Wisdom

Table 4.1: Outline of Erikson's psychosocial developmental theory

Activity 4.5 — *Critical thinking*

In Activity 4.2 you considered the physiological changes occurring for an adolescent. Alongside these, Erikson identifies a psychosocial crisis that they will be trying to resolve. What will you need to take into consideration in your care of them?

There is an outline answer at the end of the chapter.

Recognition of the psychosocial stage of the person will help guide you about what crisis they are attempting to balance and their environmental needs. For example, if a person is in middle adulthood, they need an environment in which they can show care for others. If they are denied the opportunity to show care, they may stagnate and withdraw from society, which will reduce their ability to manage older age and death with integrity and without despair.

Other significant theories developed from the psychodynamic approach are the attachment theories. John Bowlby (1907–1990) developed the theory of attachment from his work as a child psychiatrist, from psychodynamic theory and from **ethology**. Attachment theorists identify a critical period for developing attachment with the primary caregiver, which has a long-lasting impact on the child. Attachment, a close intimate bond between caregiver and child, occurs usually between the ages of eight and 12 months. Bowlby said that this attachment facilitates the development of an internal working model of what the world is like. If the child can develop a strong attachment with their caregiver, they develop a model that relationships can be based on trust and that the world is generally a benevolent place. This can clearly be seen to correspond with Erikson's stage 1.

If a child does not develop an attachment or attachments with their caregiver, they may believe the world is an untrustworthy place and that danger lurks around each corner. The attachment theorists have found that this can lead to social deviance and mental illness.

These differing psychodynamic theories offer us as nurses a unique way in which to understand, interact with and help people throughout their lifespan.

Humanistic psychology

The humanists consider themselves to be the third force in psychology after the behaviourists and psychodynamic theorists. They seek to find the humanness of the person, their uniqueness, rather than a position on a trait continuum (biological) or generalised responses to the environment (behavioural). They do not see people as purely victims of their physical bodies and competing internal and external forces (psychodynamic), although they recognise these are important. They identify that people have the power to control their experiences and behaviour.

The humanist psychologists do not offer a developmental theory, as with the behaviourists, but give nurses a view of the person that is both positive and optimistic, recognising that although each person is unique, they all have similar needs. Carl Rogers (1951) provides a complex explanation of a person's self-concept involving the 'I' and the 'me'. The 'I' is the part of ourselves we show others and the 'me' is what we know about ourselves; we can have conscious awareness of both of these. Using these elements of our personality, we try to promote an idealised view of ourselves (ideal self) with an understanding of what we are actually like (actual self). If our ideal self and actual self are similar, we will have high self-esteem; if they are far apart, we will suffer low self-esteem.

Case study: David Candiah

David was self-employed as an electrician until he retired. When he retired he became a volunteer driver for the local hospital. He enjoyed this because it not only made him feel useful – he had an important role in society – but it also gave him the opportunity to chat to a number of different people during the week. He had been having memory problems and been irritable with his partner who had persuaded him to see his GP. This led eventually to a diagnosis of Alzheimer's dementia. He has now been told that he will need to stop driving.

Activity 4.6   *Critical thinking*

Given your understanding from the humanistic approach, how might the situation affect David's self-esteem? How could you help David?

An outline answer can be found at the end of the chapter.

The humanists identify **self-actualisation** as the goal of living for humans; this can be achieved through need fulfilment and being true to oneself. For Rogers, all people need non-judgemental positive regard, which early in life is provided by the child's parents through unconditional love. Self-actualisation occurs when the person achieves their potential in whatever they are doing. This is sometimes referred to as a peak experience. The humanists see the person as having control and choice over their experiences and behaviour, and the person as always developing; self-actualisation is never completed or finished.

Self-esteem – how a person feels about themselves – is a key element of personality for the humanists. People's feelings of self-worth vary considerably over short periods of time, but self-esteem is a fairly stable construct. Terry Pratchett (2008), on hearing he was diagnosed with dementia, said:

> *When in* Paradise Lost *Milton's Satan stood in the pit of hell and raged at heaven, he was merely a trifle miffed compared to how I felt that day. I felt totally alone, with the world receding from me in every direction and you could have used my anger to weld steel.*

Despite this overwhelming sense of anger, Pratchett has gone on to campaign and promote research and care for people with this diagnosis, which will enhance his self-esteem.

The standard model of dementia is that the person changes; their personality is different after developing the condition. Given the differing psychological theories of personality above, we may be able to offer a different view. We may suggest that the person's behaviours – what we see of their personality – have changed due to previous and current learning of how to cope with difficult situations to fulfil their needs. Read the case study of Emily Stuart; the different psychological approaches can offer you a number of views of how Emily is experiencing the world.

Case study: Emily Stuart

Emily is 80 years old and had been a school teacher for 45 years in a primary school. She was respected by her colleagues and dedicated her life to the education of young children. She had always been a smartly dressed woman, and she lived in the small cottage that had belonged to her parents before their death. She had lived with her parents all her life and at the end of their lives had cared for them. The house was small but sufficient, and Emily kept it and the small garden well tended. When she retired from teaching she found that her memory deteriorated, but she developed strategies to manage with this cognitive impairment. She kept herself active by going into the school each week as a volunteer, from which she gained a lot of pleasure.

When Emily reached 75, she stopped volunteering as it was making her very tired, and she slowly reduced most of her other social interactions such as attending the Women's Institute. She noticed that her memory was becoming more of a problem as she occasionally got lost when out shopping, but there was always someone in her village to subtly guide her back home. She also noticed that she was developing urinary incontinence.

Emily's neighbour became concerned about her because she was no longer caring for her garden as she used to, and she asked Emily if she would like her son to help. Given this opportunity, Emily explained her concerns. Her neighbour contacted the Alzheimer's Society with Emily's permission. A person from the Society came to visit Emily and her neighbour, and recommended speaking to Emily's GP to get a diagnosis and support. The person explained that there might be many reasons for Emily's experiences.

After a few routine tests, the GP referred Emily to the memory clinic where she was assessed and diagnosed with Alzheimer's dementia. Emily's neighbour went along with her to the clinic to support her. The nurses at the memory clinic discussed with Emily and her neighbour how she could be supported. They asked Emily if she was happy for her neighbour to be identified as her next of kin and carer as Emily was assessed as having capacity to make this decision. After explaining the condition Emily had and its likely progression, the neighbour still wanted to offer Emily the support she needed.

continued . . .

The nurses recognised that Emily and her neighbour were managing very well but felt that some medication would be helpful. Emily was prescribed Aricept (donepezil hydrochloride); the pharmacist organised the medication into a dispensing box, and her neighbour checked that Emily was taking it at the right time. Emily and her neighbour were managing well with the support from the nurse at the memory clinic and from the Alzheimer's Society.

Activity 4.7 — Critical thinking

How can the different psychological approaches help you understand Emily's **lifeworld** experiences? How may this influence your care?

An outline answer is given at the end of the chapter.

The differing psychological approaches can be used together by nurses to help them to understand how the person may experience their world and respond to it. The approaches are philosophically different: the biological and psychodynamic theorists indicate that the person is born with certain abilities, needs and desires, while the behaviourists, cognitivists and humanists focus on how they become who they are after birth. The environment is significant for all of them.

It is recognised that it is important to listen to the lifeworld experiences of people with dementia. The lifeworld consists of the totality of their experience, their perceptions, feelings, interactions, social and political status and how they gain meaning from their world. Despite this, there is little research that has been conducted with them, and most of the research that has been undertaken is on the early stages of dementia (Morris and Morris, 2010). From the information that is available, a significant experience is one of loss: loss of self-identity, occupation, independence and companionship, which can lead to isolation, depression, low self-esteem and poor confidence (Morris and Morris, 2010).

As nurses, recognition that a person with dementia may experience these feelings can guide us to support the maintenance of self-identity, occupation, independence and companionship. These are integral to a person-centred humanised approach to care highlighted throughout this book and explored further in Chapter 7.

Alongside the individual concerns of self-identity, occupation and independence, people need companionship. They do not exist in a vacuum – they are in relationship with others. Relationship with others is an important factor in person-centred care, and Kitwood (1997) labelled this 'personhood'.

Personhood

Personhood can be seen to be the central concept in Kitwood's person-centred care. He defines it as *a standing or status that is bestowed on one human being, by another, in the context of relationship and social being* (Kitwood, 1997, p8). Kitwood believes that providing personhood facilitates the person with dementia to be valued and treated with respect. The lifeworld experiences for the person with dementia can be divided into three categories: personal characteristics; associated health status; and affiliation (Morris and Morris, 2010).

- Personal characteristics – outlook, personality, education.
- Associated health statuses – type and nature of dementia, disability, other conditions.
- Affiliation – groups a person belongs to; for example, culture, age, gender, family.

We considered personal characteristics earlier in this chapter and health status will be considered in Chapter 6. The rest of this chapter will therefore consider the elements of affiliation that were not discussed in Chapter 3.

The groups that a person is affiliated to can be quite diverse, but the primary affiliation for most people in the UK is the group they consider to be their family. Family members are usually related by blood or marriage, but can also consist of others they have an intimate relationship with. Through this family the person can gain a sense of belonging, essential for the maintenance of health according to Maslow (Barker, 2007), attachment and inclusion needs identified by Kitwood (1997) and togetherness according to Todres et al. (2009).

The family can provide for the needs of the person with dementia in ways that we, as nurses, cannot, which means that we need to view the family's needs and experiences as extremely important. This has been recognised within the National Dementia Strategy (DH, 2009), and policy and legislation has been put into place to support the family as they care for the person. The *Carers and Disabled Children Act 2000 and Carers (Equal Opportunities) Act 2004 combined policy guidance* (DH, 2004) sets out the obligation of health and social services to provide an assessment of the needs of carers and appropriate care for them.

To support the family caring for the person with dementia we need to understand their experiences. Experiences of caring for a family member with dementia can be quite diverse, but for most there are personal struggles involved. During Carers Week in 2011 Dementia UK highlighted some of these experiences using a variety of media, and on their website can be found descriptions of the feeling of some carers (Dementia UK, 2011).

Helen said, *Caring can become a very lonely existence and it has taken real effort to create a life for myself aside from spending time every day with Geoff.* David explained the impact of caring for his wife with dementia:

> One day I realised I couldn't cope any more and, arriving at work, I looked at my desk and thought: 'If I sit down there I am just going to start screaming.' I was off work for 6 months but was then able to go back to work part-time, which gave me time to do the housework and shopping. However, in 2007 it became unsafe to leave Joan on her own, so I gave up my job to become a full-time 24/7 carer.

Manjit also struggled but found some of the services helpful: *Day Care became very important to me because I was working full time and I was worried about Dad's safety as he wandered around the streets of Wolverhampton* (Dementia UK, 2011).

While there are many struggles for people caring for their family members with dementia, it is usually something they say they need to do, not just because they feel morally obliged but because they also gain pleasure in the person's company and have the opportunity to show their love for them. It is often a traumatic experience when they can no longer manage and have to release their relative to be cared for by others – see the case study of Joshua Moore.

Case study: Joshua Moore

Joshua had a close relationship with his wife, and when she developed dementia in her fifties he gave up his job to look after her. This led to reduced finances, but he wanted to spend as much time as possible with her to enjoy what interactions they could achieve. She slowly needed more personal care, and he gradually had to adapt his home and his life to incorporate hoists and wheelchairs. He found bathing and toileting his wife uncomfortable at first, but over time became accustomed to this. When she started to become agitated at night, waking the neighbours, Joshua realised that he could no longer give her the care she needed at home. It was a heart-breaking decision for him to place her in a nursing home. Joshua visited her for several hours every day at the nursing home and gradually realised he could enjoy her company again, instead of spending all his time and energy just 'getting by', doing the necessary chores and tasks. He could now spend time looking at photographs with her and reading to her. He felt he could once again have a meaningful relationship with her.

Nursing a person with dementia involves understanding how they experience what is happening to them; it is a unique experience despite the similarities between people. To best care for a person with dementia we need also to consider the experiences of their family, their carers, and these are also unique. While some people are unable to offer the care Joshua was able to, some will also not be able to release their family member into the care of others.

Chapter summary

This chapter has considered what it means to be a person and how people develop and change throughout the lifespan using the five psychological perspectives: biological, behavioural, cognitive, psychodynamic and humanistic. These approaches offer nurses an understanding of how a person might experience the world. The humanistic approach guides us to acknowledge people as unique individuals but in relationships with others. This approach underpins Kitwood's personhood and Todres et al.'s humanised care. This guides us to seek an understanding of the experiences of not only the individual with dementia but also their family and their caregivers.

Activities: brief outline answers

Activity 4.2: Critical thinking (page 65)

- Growth spurt – can cause lack of coordination and proneness to accidents.
- Myelination and synaptic growth increases – restructuring of the brain, particularly in the visuospatial and executive function (planning and self-control) areas and speeding of nervous impulses – may mean problems with planning and self-control until adolescence is concluded.

- Boys' increase in muscle growth and lung capacity – may lead to competitive relationships.
- Girls' increase in body fat – may lead to embarrassment.
- Sex-related changes – may wish to hide their changing body shape; hormones can have an impact on cognitive functioning, particularly spatial and verbal abilities.

Activity 4.4: Critical thinking (page 67)

As Elsie has low self-efficacy, she already believes she has little control over her life and has been dependent on her husband; with this diagnosis she may become more dependent. As her nurse, your main role will be to identify what her strengths are and reinforce them to facilitate her understanding that she does have control over her environment and her life despite her diagnosis.

Activity 4.5: Critical thinking (page 70)

Psychosocial crisis at this stage is identity versus identity confusion. Establishing an identity allows the person to recognise not only who they are but also who they are going to be. If this is not achieved, the person will have role confusion, which creates problems with intimacy, sense of time (ability to plan ahead), commitment (industry) and delinquency. As a nurse, you can support the young person by identifying their strengths and interests with them, recognising their effort and commitment, and by offering them positive regard.

Activity 4.6: Critical thinking (page 71)

David's self-esteem may become low as his actual self is becoming further away from his ideal self. He enjoyed being useful and people recognising him as having an important role. You need to recognise this change as being difficult for David, and respect and validate his feelings, but you also need to work with him to help him find other ways to gain the social engagement he enjoys and to maintain a helping role in a way that does not involve driving. He could perhaps volunteer as a befriender and visit people who cannot leave their homes.

Activity 4.7: Critical thinking (page 73)

Biological: As Emily has aged, it is likely that plaques and tangles will have occurred in her brain, causing brain cell death. This may not have had any impact on Emily's behaviour due to neural plasticity, but we can see that Emily has developed dementia, so the brain cell death is having an impact on her experiences. Her muscles and bones will have reduced in size, and her senses, such as sight and hearing, will be less effective. Emily's personality traits should remain the same, but some of her behaviours may change to cope with her physiological changes. These changes should be in keeping with her personality unless there is extensive brain cell death in the fronto-temporal cortex. She may need your help to understand this and why she needs to take the prescribed medication.

Behaviourist: The behaviourists would suggest she has learnt to behave in certain ways – become the person she is – because of associations and reinforced behaviours. Her lifeworld experiences are due to the environment in which she finds herself. Emily learnt to be independent and care for others, so when she started to have problems she did not seek help. Her self-efficacy could initially be seen to be high as she appears to believe she can manage her symptoms by changing her environment herself. Her self-efficacy may now have diminished as she has had to seek help and this will increase as her condition becomes worse. This can be reduced by others such as her neighbour and the nurse helping her to make as many choices about her future as possible so she feels she has some control.

Cognitive: The cognitive psychologists would identify that Emily has learnt to be who she is but that this is not without cognitive processing. Emily would have learnt not only from association and reward, but also through observing others. In these ways she will have determined how she would like to behave and live her life. As her memory has declined she will have depended on her intelligence and problems-solving abilities to adapt. As she has aged, these will be based on experiential abilities – crystallised intelligence and intuitive problem solving – but dementia will reduce her ability to do this. As a nurse you will need to support her continued use of her abilities by maintaining them through reminiscent therapy and by encouraging her to think about how she would like to manage any problems that occur.

Psychodynamic/psychosocial: Using Erikson's theory, it may be assumed that Emily may have problems with middle and late adulthood, as she never completed the crisis of young adulthood as she has remained single throughout her life. It would appear, though, that Emily has addressed the crisis of middle life by caring for and nurturing children in school. It may also be that she has gained love through her relationships with her parents, at school, in her social group or with neighbours. If this is the case, Emily should have a strong ego and have faced late adulthood with the ability to balance the crisis of integrity versus despair. Her experience of dementia may, though, affect her sense of person integrity as symptoms increase and could lead to despair rather than wisdom. Using a person-centred and humanising approach will help Emily to retain her sense of herself as a person and retain integrity, facilitating the achievement of wisdom and acceptance of herself and others.

Humanist: Emily would appear to have gained positive regard throughout her life through her parents, colleagues and children at school and her neighbours. This will have facilitated her meeting her maintenance and development needs. She has exhibited control and choice in her life, and her ideal and actual selves appear to have been close together, indicating high self-esteem. Using the humanistic approach, though, it is only Emily who can say whether these things are true; it is Emily's understanding of her world that is important. Her ideal self appears to be an independent, caring and capable person; the advent of dementia has reduced her independence and her ability to care for others. This may cause a gulf between her actual and ideal self and create low self-esteem. You will need to support Emily's independence and help her find ways to continue to show her care for others to maintain her self-esteem and her sense of well-being.

Further reading

Adams, T (2008) *Dementia care nursing: promoting well-being in people with dementia and their families.* Basingstoke: Palgrave Macmillan.

This book considers the areas of the personal and family experiences of dementia in more detail. It offers a strong theoretical and research base.

Barker, S (2007) *Vital notes for nurses: psychology.* Oxford: Blackwell.

This book offers a clear and concise overview of the psychological theories that underpin nursing practice, and more detail and case studies related to lifespan development.

Useful websites

http://guidance.nice.org.uk/CG42

The National Institute for Health and Clinical Excellence is a government body that provides guidance for many sorts of health issues. This particular guidance (CG42) is *Dementia: supporting people with dementia and their carers in health and social care.*

www.dementiauk.org

Dementia UK is a dementia charity that has lots of useful information on their website. You can access some of the personal experiences of family members who are caring for a relative who has dementia. A direct link to carers' experiences is also provided at: **www.dementiauk.org/get-involved/carers-week/carers-experiences**.

Chapter 5
Nursing assessment

continued . . . •••

By entry to the register:

xii. In partnership with the person, their carers and their families, makes a holistic, person-centred and systematic assessment of physical, emotional, psychological, social, cultural and spiritual needs, including risk, and together, develops a comprehensive personalised plan of nursing care.

xiii. Acts autonomously and takes responsibility for collaborative assessment and planning of care delivery with the person, their carers and their family.

Chapter aims

On completion of this chapter you should have developed an understanding of:

- the scope of dementia care assessment;
- the differences between delirium and dementia;
- holistic nursing assessment.

Introduction

The number of people with dementia is expected to increase exponentially in the future, and new treatments are becoming available. Because of this, the government has led initiatives to improve recognition of dementia in the early stages of the disease. Following the introduction of the Dementia Care Strategy (DH, 2009), aimed at health professionals such as nurses, in 2011 the government started a £2 million campaign to raise awareness among the general public. Through leaflets, radio and TV advertisements, this campaign encouraged people to recognise the early signs of dementia and go to the doctor. This chapter will explore how an assessment of dementia nursing care is made. Using a case study, it will illustrate how a person with dementia may present in a variety of care environments and the nurses' role in their care within a multi-disciplinary team.

Nursing assessment

Ebersole and Hess (1998) quote Daisy, aged 82, who discusses how her grandfather used to assess his patients: *You know, in the old days when my grandfather was practising he would diagnose by sight, feel, smell, and taste. Yes taste! But of course, nobody ever heard of a malpractice suit either.*

A comprehensive nursing assessment is essential for all the care we provide. According to the NMC (2010a), it is one of the necessary competencies to practise as a registered nurse. The NMC offers a clear expectation of a nurse's assessment in the essential skills clusters for registered nurses (see above). This includes a holistic assessment that takes account of relevant physical, social, cultural, psychological, spiritual, genetic and environmental factors. The assessment should be conducted in partnership with the interprofessional team, the person concerned, their carers and their family. This is especially relevant when assessing an individual who is **cognitively challenged** and has problems organising their thinking. While a person-centred approach is important in all areas of nursing, it is crucial to understand the experience of a person with dementia: who they are; their problems with living their life in a way they would choose; and the abilities and skills they have at the point when a diagnosis of dementia is suspected.

There are a number of approaches that nurses can use to conduct their assessments. These include:

- an interview with the person, their carer and family, using a semi-structured interview or a storytelling approach;
- questionnaires and rating scales that measure consciousness, cognitive skills, mood, anxiety, and so on; there are a number of these available to nurses;
- direct observation, including noting clinical signs in the eyes, skin, nails, etc. and measuring blood pressure and fluid intake.

There are a number of nursing models that support a holistic nursing assessment – you can read about them in Chapter 2. There are also two interprofessional assessment processes used in mental health services – the Single Assessment Approach and the Care Programme Approach – but these do not tend to be used by other areas. Most assessment processes appear to focus on problems, but the models developed by Kitwood (1993), Nolan et al. (2004) and Todres et al. (2009) encourage the assessment of dementia care to be focused on strengths. To undertake any assessment you need to be able to communicate effectively with everyone involved, so it is communication that we now discuss.

Communication

Communication is central to a nurse's role. If you cannot communicate with others, you cannot nurse. This means that you need to demonstrate the ability to listen, attend and respond. Core communication skills necessary for nurses can be found in the psychological literature and are widely used throughout health and social care. Carl Rogers (1951) outlined the core attitudes and skills to develop and maintain effective communication.

- Respecting the person.
- Being genuine, trusting, sincere and honest.
- Being good at listening, attending and responding.
- Accepting the person unconditionally.
- Showing empathy.
- Being non-judgemental.

Gerard Egan went on to establish an approach to communication in helping relationships. He gave some concrete guidance on this by outlining interviewing techniques that will help you collect information for assessment, under the acronym SOLER.

S – Sit squarely; upright and alert.

O – Open posture; uncrossed arms and legs.

L – Lean forward; but not to the extent of invading their personal space.

E – Eye contact; maintain eye contact but do not stare.

R – Relax; this will demonstrate confidence.

Egan also gave detailed guidance on verbal and non-verbal communication. To facilitate verbal interaction you could incorporate the appropriate use of open and closed questions, reflecting, paraphrasing, echoing and summarising in your assessments. Non-verbally, you could respond to people through postural echo, nodding, smiling, touch and silence, all of which are powerful when used at the right time.

Activity 5.1   *Communication*

Think of a time when you were communicating with a person you were caring for. Try to remember whether you used the **SOLER** techniques. Make a note of how you could improve.

With a friend, try out using the non-verbal responses mentioned above. Take turns to explore a personal issue, one asking questions and using the non-verbal responses.

How did it feel? The more you practise with these the easier they will become.

As this is a personal reflection, there is no outline answer at the end of the chapter.

Communication skills are essential in nursing but particularly so when nursing people who have dementia, as their sensory perception may be limited and frequently their ability to communicate with you may be impaired.

Assessment of dementia care is not a short process; it can be seen more in terms of a journey. The case study of Brenda Drake will help you to start to explore the journey towards a nursing assessment.

Case study: Mrs Brenda Drake – Part 1

Brenda lives with her husband Bob in a semi-detached house they bought when they were first married 60 years ago. They have four children and nine grandchildren. Brenda and Bob are very family orientated and enjoy spending time with their family. In the past they played a key role in the child care of their grandchildren while their parents worked. This was a role that both Brenda and Bob found very fulfilling. Brenda enjoys cooking, knitting, reading and watching dramas on the television. Bob spends a great deal of time maintaining his garden, and enjoys watching the soaps in the evening. Bob continues to drive but only short journeys to the shops and the cliff top for weekly walks by the sea. Each Christmas Brenda and Bob invite their family over for a meal and party games. Brenda prepares an abundance of food: her children laugh at her as she serves yet another plate of vol-au-vents. This is a family standing joke that secretly Brenda enjoys. Two years ago, as

---

continued . . .

> *Brenda's daughter and her family arrive for the Christmas get-together, Brenda grabs her daughter and whisks her off to the kitchen. Brenda appears very anxious and asks her daughter to take over in the kitchen. The kitchen is chaotic, with cupboards open and the sink full of dirty crockery. Brenda is normally a very organised and tidy cook. She says that she feels disorganised and not on 'top of it all'. The meal is almost ready, and Brenda with her daughter's assistance serves it to the rest of the family.*

Activity 5.2   *Critical thinking*

Take a few minutes to consider Brenda's behaviour and make notes on what you think about it. There could be many reasons why she is very anxious and does not appear as organised as normal. What might they be?

There is an outline answer at the end of the chapter.

As this book is about dementia, you would be correct in thinking that Brenda may be showing early signs of dementia. The symptoms of dementia may present many years before a formal diagnosis is made. Loss of concentration and an inability to organise familiar tasks may be early signs. However, people and their families may dismiss these signs, saying they are part of getting old. People will often disguise their problems and adapt their behaviour to meet the challenges they face when experiencing symptoms of dementia. Families may see changes when there is a long gap between visits, and subtle symptoms can be observed with fresh eyes. The Department of Health document *Living well with dementia* (DH, 2009) emphasises the importance of early diagnosis to ensure people have access to appropriate support: *The evidence available . . .points strongly to the value of early diagnosis and intervention to improve quality of life and to delay or prevent unnecessary admissions into care homes* (DH, 2009, p34).

In November 2011 the Department of Health started a new campaign to raise awareness of the early signs and symptoms of dementia. It aims to encourage more people to seek an early diagnosis. The campaign targets the family and friends of people at risk of dementia who are most likely to be the first to see the signs and encourage their loved one to see their GP. An early diagnosis can help people with dementia get the right treatment and support, and help those close to them to prepare and plan for the future. With treatment and support, many people are able to lead active, fulfilling lives. The TV advert tells the story of the daughter as she becomes aware that her father is struggling in a number of situations, such as leaving pans on the hob of the cooker and forgetting where his car is parked. While the advert makes it clear that it was a hard issue to raise, the message is that acting on her concerns and getting help means that the daughter can keep 'the father she knows' for longer.

Nurses in all care settings must be aware of their role in promoting health and encourage people to seek medical advice when their health deviates from their normal. The *Common core principles for supporting people with dementia* document (DH, 2011a) outlines in Principle 1 the early signs of dementia that health care workers such as nurses need know. These are:

- loss or lapses of recent memory;
- mood changes or uncharacteristic behaviour;
- poor concentration;
- problems communicating;
- getting lost in familiar places;
- making mistakes in a previously learnt skill;
- problems telling the time or using money;
- changes in sleep patterns and appetite;
- personality changes;
- **visuospatial** perception issues.

If you recognise any of these signs, you need to encourage the person to seek further assessment. Appropriate assessment is key, not only to diagnosis if a person has a dementia but also to identify any other underlying pathology.

Activity 5.3   *Evidence-based practice and research*

Take a few minutes to consider a patient or relative that you have cared for who has a diagnosis of dementia. Note down how they appeared to you. How would you describe their presenting features? Consider the presenting features of dementia and how you might notice these in practice.

An outline answer is given at the end of the chapter.

Features associated with dementia

While considering, in Activity 5.3, how dementia may present itself, you may have noted confusion, memory difficulties, repetition of words or sentences or requests, disorientation, anxiety or even aggression. These symptoms can be easily dismissed as the ageing process or attributed to dementia with the belief that nothing further can be done.

There is a danger that without a comprehensive **multi-dimensional** assessment, dementia and other diseases such as depression or a delirium may go untreated. Even when a diagnosis of dementia is made, there is much that nurses can do, in collaboration with the person and others, to improve the quality of life and well-being for the person and their family. Chapter 7 explores care options.

The various clinical features that are attributed to dementia have many overlaps with the clinical features of depression or an acute confusion/delirium. For example, people with any one of these conditions may be disorientated, anxious or forgetful, and have a fluctuating level of cognition affecting their memory, orientation and attention. The person may even present with one, two or even three of these conditions at the same time. The skill of nurses and the **inter-disciplinary** team is needed to undertake a comprehensive assessment. The nurse's role is key both in the contribution to the assessment but also the coordination of the team.

Foreman (1996) distinguished between the clinical features of depression, dementia and acute confusion/delirium, and these are displayed in Table 5.1. A notable feature of delirium is its acute

Elements	Delirium	Depression	Dementia
Onset	Occurs in the evening	May be rapid after a traumatic event or slow where there is no trauma	Slow onset
Features	Worse in evening, dark and early morning	Worse in morning	Even throughout day
Development	Abrupt start	Slow or rapid start but even progression	Slow start and uneven progression
Length	Less than a month	Over two weeks	Months to years
Awareness	Unaware	Aware	Aware
Attention	Impaired	Varies	Normal
Alertness	Low or high	Normal	Normal
Orientation	Impaired	Varies	Varies
Thinking	Impaired, speech affected	Focus on negative, hopelessness	Impaired
Memory	Recent impaired	Varies	Recent and remote impaired
Perception	Grossly distorted	Normal unless severe	Normal but some variation
Motor skills	Impaired	Varies – agitation or slowness may occur	Normal
Sleep	Disturbed	Early morning wakening	Fragmented
Response to mental tests	Grossly impaired	Lacks interest and motivation	Impaired – struggles to answer
Other	Associated with physical health problem, mood swings and personality exaggerated	Low mood, negative thoughts, preoccupation with self	Rapid mood swings, difficulty finding words, offers explanations for inability.

Table 5.1: Comparing delirium, depression and dementia

Source: adapted from Foreman (1996).

Note: The table provides the usual or more common elements of the three conditions, but in different types of depression and dementia these may vary.

onset; people will have experienced a sudden deterioration of their cognition over a short period. With dementia, the patient will have experienced a more gradual decline; while depression may be **insidious,** developing slowly and frequently coinciding with a specific life event.

Acute confusion/delirium

Acute confusion or delirium is characterised by disorganised thinking, a decreased attention span, fluctuating consciousness, disturbance in the sleep–wake cycle, disorientation, and changes in psycho-motor skills (Henry, 2002). Unlike dementia, delirium has an acute onset, and, if treated appropriately, is reversible.

From a personal and family perspective, timely comprehensive assessment of confusion is vital. The consequences of delirium not being diagnosed are significant. The risk of **mortality** – dying as an outcome of this physical health problem – increases from between 22 per cent to 76 per cent. The length of stay in hospital is likely to increase, so the chances of falls and of developing pressure sores, pneumonia or hospital-acquired infection also increase. Those who survive undiagnosed delirium are more likely to be transferred to long-term care with a decline in both **functional** and cognitive status. This has a subsequent financial cost for both health and social care providers.

In 2007 the charity Age Concern launched a campaign to raise awareness of the assessment and management of delirium. It emphasised that acute confusion is a sign that someone is physically unwell and identifies a three-point plan for the assessment and management of delirium: Spot it, Treat it, Stop it.

Spotting delirium can be a challenge. The literature identifies three types of delirium: **hyperactive**, **hypoactive** and mixed. Hyperactive delirium is characterised by restlessness, agitation and irritability, and may include **hallucinations**. In contrast, the hypoactive form **manifests** itself as withdrawal, apathy, lethargy and decreased psycho-motor activity. This latter form is difficult to recognise because the person may be assumed to be compliant and contented. Fluctuations can also occur between hyperactivity and hypoactivity.

Clinical features of delirium are characterised by a sudden change in behaviour. This change may have occurred over a few hours or days. The person may present as more confused than normal. Confusion may fluctuate in severity but is usually worse at night, often made worse by poor light.

Theory summary: confusion assessment

The confusion assessment method is a quick tool used in identifying confusion. A comprehensive nursing assessment is indicated if features 1 and 2 and 3 or 4 in the list are present.

1. Acute onset and fluctuating course.
2. Inattention.
3. Disorganised thinking.
4. Altered level of consciousness.

An **acute confusional state** is usually assessed in acute hospital settings.

Nursing assessment in the acute setting

A patient admitted into the acute general hospital setting presenting with a history of confusion and memory problems needs a comprehensive assessment to identify the cause of the symptoms. Let us return to Brenda's case study. You will recall from Part 1 of the case study that Brenda had had problems with organising her usual Christmas meal for her family; her condition continues to deteriorate.

Case study: Mrs Brenda Drake – Part 2

Brenda, with the encouragement of her family, goes to see her GP who contacts the local district general hospital. Brenda is admitted, via the accident and emergency department, to an acute medical ward. The letter from Mrs Drake's GP states that she has become confused and disorientated over the last few days. She has been reluctant to get washed and dressed and has refused the assistance of her husband. She has been incontinent of urine and does not appear to notice this. Mr Drake is very anxious and is struggling to cope.

On admission to the ward the following observations are recorded.

- *Temperature 37.2° Celsius.*
- *Pulse 100 beats per minute, irregular, thready.*
- *Blood pressure reading systolic 170mmhg (millimetres of mercury) and diastolic 95mmhg.*
- *Blood oxygen saturation 96%.*

Her husband provides the following information on her past medical history.

- *Hysterectomy eight years ago.*
- *Occasional paracetamol for headaches.*

Activity 5.4   *Critical thinking*

As the nurse on duty, how would you begin the assessment of Brenda? In undertaking an assessment of Brenda you may well take into account her chronological age. The normal range for the measurements taken will vary according to age. Use the confusion assessment method to assess whether she may have delirium. What are your reasons for your answer?

An outline answer in provided at the end of the chapter.

Age Concern, which developed the Spot it, Treat it, Stop it campaign for delirium, also developed an assessment strategy for it (Age Concern, 2007). It suggests that when undertaking a comprehensive assessment of a patient admitted with confusion it is important to consider what may have caused the confusion. The acronym PINCH ME reminds nurses of the many reasons for confusion and what to assess for. So when you are assessing for confusion, remember PINCH ME.

Pain

IN-fection

Constipation

Hydration

Medication

Environment

If it is decided that Brenda has delirium, she will receive the appropriate medical treatment and nursing. If she is considered to be at risk of dementia, she will need further assessment.

Assessing dementia care needs

While the focus in this section is on the role of the nursing assessment, the evidence suggests that a comprehensive assessment is essential. This is a multi-dimensional, interdisciplinary diagnostic process to determine the medical, psychological, social, spiritual and functional capabilities of the person in order to develop a coordinated and integrated plan for treatment and long-term follow-up.

As a nurse completing an assessment, you will need to bear in mind the NMC definition of assessment discussed at the beginning of the chapter. Comprehensive interprofessional assessment is crucial in identifying the cause of confusion and, when appropriate, identifying dementia.

A comprehensive assessment will involve all these aspects.

- Physical
- Psychological
- Emotional
- Environmental
- Cultural
- Social
- Spiritual

Various elements in each of these aspects will be assessed, and we will look at these next. It is also crucial that you bear in mind the risks associated with any areas of need you identify. A key concern in all areas of health care is risk assessment and risk management, and this is particularly important in dementia care. We undertake risk assessments in our lives all the time, such as whether it is safe to cross the road, but when we are caring for others we need to also assess their ability to manage their own risks, to keep themselves safe and well. For each of the areas above, as part of our assessment, we need to ask ourselves whether this is something that the person can manage themselves or whether we need to intervene. For example, if we identify that the person has a sight deficit but that they manage this by adequate lighting and by holding onto hand rails in the toilets and down the stairs, they can be assessed as low risk. On the other hand, if a person is assessed as having a sight deficit that they do not acknowledge, they may be at risk of not seeing warning signs or tripping over and falling.

Physical assessment

Respiration

By undertaking a detailed respiratory (breathing) assessment you could discover signs of a chest infection. By observing your patient you could note their facial expressions. Do they appear to be struggling when breathing? Are they using their accessory muscles? Note the colour of their skin and its condition. Is there any sign of peripheral or central **cyanosis**, which could indicate respiratory distress? It is important to notice their level of consciousness, as **cerebral hypoxia** can cause drowsiness, irritability and restlessness. Respiratory rate is also important as it can indicate that a person is struggling to get enough oxygen into their body or that they are extremely anxious; a raised respiratory rate is called tachypnoea. You should also look out for noisy breathing, as it may be an indication of bronchitis. Any problems with breathing may be a cause of delirium.

Urine

Urine testing can give an indication of many physical health problems that may trigger delirium. Collecting a routine specimen of urine (RSU) and testing using a urine test strip may indicate signs of diabetes or a urinary tract infection (UTI). Fishy odour and protein in the urine can indicate a UTI.

Constipation

It is important to ask about constipation as it can cause acute confusion due to the build-up of toxins in the body. It can also lead to physical pain and hallucinations.

Pulse and blood pressure recording

The observations from the accident and emergency department have indicated that Brenda's pulse is fast and thready and that her blood pressure is slightly elevated. While these need to be measured again, the fast and thready pulse may be an indication of **atrial fibrillation** (AF). Both AF and **hypertension** increase the risk of stroke and therefore also the risk of vascular dementia (the different types of dementia will be described in Chapter 6).

Pain

Pain can cause disorientation and confusion. The Abbey pain scale is useful for assessing pain in a confused patient (RCP, 2007). This scale involves assessment of:

- vocalisations – such as crying;
- facial expression – such as grimacing;
- change of body language – such as holding parts of the body;
- behavioural change – such as refusing to eat;
- physiological change – such as blood pressure;
- physical changes – such as skin tears.

Nutrition

A person can manage without food for some time, but if they do not have enough to drink they will quickly become dehydrated, which can lead to toxicity and confusion. You need to see if they appear dehydrated; observe skin **turgor**. When pinched around the upper chest, does the skin rebound quickly? Fluid intake and output need to be monitored, which can be done using a fluid balance chart. Care is explored in Chapter 7.

Medication review

It is important to record all the medication that Brenda is taking at home. The next of kin or carers should be asked to bring all medication in if Brenda has not arrived with them. **Polypharmacy** and certain medications such as **antidepressants** or **opiates** can cause confusion. Therefore, the medical team will need to review these as part of the multi-dimensional assessment.

Medical

The medical team will need to request further diagnostic tests; some nurses also have the authority to request these, to identify the cause of the confusion. Tests include:

- haematology;
- biochemistry;
- thyroid function;
- serum vitamin B12 and folate levels;
- chest X-rays or **electrocardiogram** (ECG).

A magnetic resonance imaging (MRI) scan may be requested to eliminate the possibility that tumours are causing the confusion, but a scan can also identify signs of vascular dementia. A special type of positron emission tomography (PET) scan may help to detect the plaques in the brain associated with Alzheimer's disease (see Chapter 6).

Activity 5.5   *Critical thinking*

What do you think the advantages and disadvantages of having a brain scan, such as an MRI, might be?

An outline answer can found at the end of the chapter.

Abnormalities revealed by any of these physical tests may mimic the symptoms of dementia, rather than actually being caused by dementia. However, if physical problems are identified and treated, they will improve the presenting symptoms.

Psychological

Mood

As was seen earlier in this chapter, depression and dementia have many similar features. Depression can be defined as an ongoing low mood that has an impact on functioning. There are a number of issues that should be considered when assessing a person's mood.

- What is normal for them? Is 'their cup usually half full or half empty'?
- Do they have a history of problems with their mood?
- Have there been some recent stressors for them, such as bereavement?
- How long have they felt like this?
- How do they cope when their feelings change?
- Do they feel like harming themselves?
- Have they felt helpless or hopeless?

These issues are mostly considered relevant to depression, but many other features that are important in assessing for depression are also implicated in delirium and dementia.

- Are they having problems with motivating themselves or being restless?
- Are they having problems sleeping or with their appetite?
- Have they had problems with attention, concentration or memory?

It is important to identify the risk factors for depression when undertaking a comprehensive assessment, as depression (as with delirium) can be life-threatening because of the risk of self-harm and suicide. A person may be suffering from depression and have dementia at the same time, so if it is decided that the person has depression, that does not rule out dementia. Depression can be treated successfully.

Cognition

Many physical and mental conditions, as well as tiredness and what has been eaten or drunk, can influence cognition, which is why it is important to consider the circumstances in which your assessment is taking place. Cognition is usually divided into attention, concentration and memory in health arenas, but problem solving is also a good area to assess functioning.

Once other conditions such as delirium and depression have been dismissed, there are numerous cognitive assessments that can be undertaken to assess functioning. The most common tool is the mini mental state examination (MMSE) developed by Folstein et al. (1975), which is not ideal for assessing people in ethnic minority groups (see Chapter 3). Despite these problems, it is the most widely used first-stage psychological assessment for people with suspected dementia and the scale is linked to prescription of dementia medications through NICE (2010). It can, though, only be used under licence from Psychological Assessment Resources (PAR). As the previous copyright holders allowed free access, it is easily found on the web. Another popular screening tool used in hospitals by nurse and occupational therapists is the revised Addenbrooke's Cognitive Examination (ACE-R) (Mioshi et al., 2006). This is longer and takes more time than the brief

MMSE or the other short cognitive impairment tests. A copy of this can be found on the web and a link is available at the end of this chapter.

There are many other short tests available that mostly consider the same areas; examples are the GP cognitive test (GP COG), the six-item cognitive impairment test (6 CIT), the abbreviated mental test (AMT) and the test your memory test (TYM). The GP COG and 6 CIT take only a small amount of time and have been found to be useful in primary care. The person is scored on how many answers they got right (Patient.co.uk, 2012).

Table 5.2 gives an overview of some of the tests available to assess cognitive impairment and an example question from each area. It is important that assessments of cognitive impairment are not made solely on these scales; as was seen in Chapter 3, there can be cultural problems with them. As nurses, we must use our comprehensive assessments and clinical judgements.

Assessment	MMSE	GP COG	6 CIT	AMT	TYM
Progress	No	Yes	No	No	No
Example	Do you have more problems remembering things now than you did last year?				
Orientation to time	Yes	Yes	Yes	Yes	Yes
Example	What is the date?				
Orientation to place	Yes	No	No	Yes	Yes
Example	Name the place we are in.				
Attention/ concentration	Yes	Not directly	Yes	Yes	Not directly
Example	Count backwards from 20.				
Memory for previous learning	Yes	Yes	No	Yes	Yes
Example	Who is the current monarch?				
Memory for new learning	Yes	Yes	Yes	Yes	Yes
Example	I want you to remember the following words and repeat them back to me in a few minutes. Pen . . . Paper . . . Bin.				

Table 5.2: Comparison of assessment using easily accessed cognitive impairment scales

Continued

Assessment	MMSE	GP COG	6 CIT	AMT	TYM
Language	Yes	Not directly	Not directly	Not directly	Yes
Example	Could you read this sentence?				
Visuospatial skills	Yes	Yes, through clock drawing	No	No	Yes
Example	Please draw the following shape: could be two geometric shapes overlapping				
Clock drawing	No	Yes	No	No	No
Example	Please draw a picture of a clock face that is showing 3 o'clock.				

Table 5.2: Continued

Perception

Perception involves an interaction between the sensory information from the environment and the brain's ability to make this meaningful. As people pass the age of 20, their sensory ability tends to decline in all the senses: hearing, sight, taste, smell, touch and **proprioception**. On the whole, the brain is quite resilient and will develop strategies to cope with this decline, and given the increased knowledge and experience collected throughout the lifespan, older people may function at a higher level than young people. See Chapter 4 for more information on psychological lifespan development.

A person's perceptual ability can be assessed using the MMSE and ACE-R. As people with dementia may have perceptual disturbances that may not be recognised in these tools, it is important that you also find out if they are having experiences such as hallucinations – unique sensual perceptions that other people do not perceive. For example, **auditory** and **visual** hallucinations are common for people who have Lewy body dementia. You can find more information on the different types of dementia in Chapter 6.

Behaviour

Behavioural 'norms' are very broad in our society, so when assessing a patient's behaviour you need to find out what is normal for them, either from them, their carer or their family. It is usually family members who notice changes and seek advice. Some of the behaviours that carers find most stressful are angry outbursts, sleep disturbance and diet changes; 'wandering' and bizarre behaviours are also reported, but these often have a significant meaning for the person concerned. Behavioural assessments can be made using the ABC model.

- Antecedent – What happened before?
- Behaviour – What are they doing?
- Consequence – What effect does it have?

If you can find out what led to the behaviour, you can more fully understand; if behavioural change is needed, the antecedent or consequence could be changed.

Activity 5.6   *Critical thinking*

You are working in a residential care setting and you find a resident apparently 'wandering' up and down the corridor untying his pyjamas. What might he think he is doing?

An outline answer is provided at the end of the chapter.

Emotional assessment

Emotions can quite rapidly fluctuate, get more or less intense, or change from one to another, and this is particularly the case for those experiencing dementia. Some of the major emotions felt by people who believe they may have dementia are anxiety and fear about the future, grief and loss, depression and loss of self-esteem, and terror. These are issues that you, as a nurse, will need to manage during the assessment process as well as after diagnosis is made (see Chapter 6). Because of these emotions, people may use coping strategies such as denial, avoidance, blaming others and covering up to protect their self-concept and self-esteem. How the person experiences their dementia will have a huge impact on their self-esteem and quality of life.

Activity 5.7   *Communication*

If you are assessing a person who is experiencing anxiety, fear, grief or low self-esteem, how could you respond to them to reduce these uncomfortable feelings?

There is an outline answer at the end of the chapter.

It is important that you are respectful and sensitive when exploring the person's experiences, as this will help them maintain their self-esteem and feelings of self-worth. If a person loses self-esteem or feelings of self-worth, they may become depressed and fail to take part in activities that promote well-being.

Environmental assessment

There are a number of elements within the environment that need to be assessed when caring for a person who may have dementia. Maslow's hierarchy of needs is a useful model (see Chapter 7 for a more detailed discussion of this model). The main question we need to ask ourselves using this model is: does the environment provide the space in which the person can fulfil their health-maintaining and developmental needs?

- Maintenance needs: physiological, safety, love and belonging, esteem.
- Developmental needs: cognitive, aesthetic, self-actualisation.

In nursing we frequently use a more simplistic approach to the environment, and the assessment areas include the following.

- Physical environment – Is the lighting adequate?
- People – Can attachment and belonging be achieved with others?
- Culture – Do the rituals and routines make sense and fit with their personal belief system?

Whichever approach is used in this assessment, the person needs to feel safe and comfortable in their environment.

Activity 5.8   *Critical thinking*

Reread Brenda's case study – Part 2. Make notes on how the hospital environment might increase Brenda's confusion and distress.

There is an outline answer at the end of the chapter.

Socio-cultural assessment

We live in a multi-cultural society. As we saw in Chapter 3, society provides the structure within which people in very large groups can organise themselves through legislation and behavioural norms. Within this structure, our own culture provides us with a belief system and the roles we need to fulfil. Much of the abnormal behaviour observed in those with dementia can be attributed to social stereotypes and the internalisation of these by the person. Due to their early socialisation, people with dementia accept the stereotypes that society holds for them and behave in a way that fulfils expectations. Within this stereotype, they are identified as worthless and incurable, which also leads them not to seek help.

When you are assessing whether a person has socio-cultural needs that require nursing support, you need to seek the understanding and experiences of the person, their carer and their family. Do not make assumptions based on your own socio-cultural background; it may be different. Find out how their family is organised and their role within it, and remember that this may change with the progression of dementia.

There are a number of areas that need exploration.

- *Living arrangements* – who they live with and how they are managing at home. Alongside this, occupational therapists (OTs) will frequently conduct specific home assessments to check, for example, safety when cooking.
- *Support network* – what support network is available; whether they live alone or with an extended family, if there are people around who can take on the role of carer.
- *Mobility* – can be a cause for concern inside and outside the home. Inside the home, is the lighting adequate? Are stairs or carpets a problem? Outside the home, can the person get to

the shops to buy their food, visit friends or get to other engagements? A structured assessment of this is frequently undertaken by OTs, but if you are visiting the home, as a nurse you need to be mindful of safety and assess for these things.

- *Financial assessment* – nurses rarely do a detailed assessment of a person's financial situation, but we need to ask questions at the assessment about whether the person has any problems in this area, and inform them that financial support may be available. With their permission, we can then refer them to other members of the multi-disciplinary team (MDT), such as a social worker, who may be able to help.
- *Legal* – there are a number of legal issues that a person with dementia needs to consider, particularly early after diagnosis, and it is important that this is raised with them as soon as possible. The Alzheimer's Society and Age UK are very helpful in guiding people through some of the decisions they may need to make, such as power of attorney. As a nurse, you may need to be involved in assessing whether a person is competent under the Mental Capacity Act to make decisions for themselves (see Chapter 8).
- *Social groups* – it is helpful for care planning to know if the person attends any type of social groups as these can provide valuable support networks; you may need to explore ways in which the person can continue to attend them.
- *Carer needs assessment* – an assessment of the carer's needs is usually undertaken by a social worker, but this is something that you should raise with the carer as they may be unaware of the support available to them. Adequate support should reduce the risk of the carer developing their own health problems.

Spiritual assessment

A person's spiritual life and belief system are crucial to their quality of life and well-being, and it is now recognised in health care that spirituality is an important area for nurses to assess (see Chapter 3). Nurses need to be aware of the wide diversity of spirituality in our society. They could initially ask questions related to religion, or focus on the broader aspects, such as asking about somewhere they go or something they do that makes them feel at peace, and feel comfortable. Nurses need to explore how the person makes sense of the world and what gives it meaning for them. How this is asked or phrased will depend on the situation and the people involved. If the person does not seem to understand or perhaps denies having a religion or a spiritual life, you could ask them about their values. Discuss what is important to them, what they would least like to lose, perhaps which events or social situations are most important for them to attend or if, when and where they need time and space to be alone.

Assessment of dementia

Undertaking an assessment in an acute in-patient setting can provide some significant evidence to support an assessment of dementia, but this sort of environment does not make for a trustworthy diagnosis. Therefore, you will need to review the assessment after discharge from hospital, or when the patient is more stable, or after the acute confusion has stabilised. Let us return to Brenda and see how her story is evolving.

Case study: Mrs Brenda Drake – Part 3

While in hospital, Brenda is found to have had a UTI, which has caused her delirium. With effective and skilled nursing care Brenda stabilises and is able to return home after five days. Brenda is much improved and returns to her functional baseline prior to the UTI. However, both she and Bob remain concerned about some residual memory lapses. While in hospital they completed a MMSE and a score of 22/30 was recorded, showing significant cognitive impairment; a diagnosis of dementia is considered.

Activity 5.9	*Critical thinking*

Brenda gained a low score on the MMSE (Folstein et al., 1975) which assesses for:

- orientation to time;
- orientation to place;
- attention/concentration;
- memory for previously learning information;
- memory for new information;
- language;
- visuospatial skills.

Her score indicates significant cognitive impairment.

What factors may have influenced this score?

An outline answer can be found at the end of the chapter.

Brenda's discharge letter to her GP advises that Brenda will be referred to the memory clinic to review her MMSE.

Assessment in the memory clinic

The overall aim of the memory clinic is to provide clients with a comprehensive assessment and, where appropriate, an early diagnosis of dementia, in line with the DH's National Dementia Strategy (DH, 2009). Comprehensive assessment is repeated once again with an MDT review. The role of the memory clinic is:

- diagnosis in the early stage of dementia to optimise independent living;
- diagnosis for unspecified/unexplained cognitive impairment/confusion;
- information, support and signposting for patients and carers aiming to maintain or improve quality of life;
- needs-specific person-centred care planning;
- retention of personhood despite reduced mental powers (Kitwood, 1997);

- provision of MDT care planning with outreach service;
- prescription of dementia drug therapy that complies with the National Institute for Health and Clinical Excellence (NICE) guidance.
- cognitive stimulation and memory strategy.

Standards of care in the memory clinic

The memory clinic provides supportive care for the person with dementia and their family from the moment of diagnosis. Such supportive care recognises the value of the person with dementia and aims to promote the well-being and autonomy of that person while also paying attention to the interests of carers. The focus is on the individual and not the diagnostic label.

A diagnostic label becomes irrelevant if the person with dementia is cared for with respect, is valued as a family member and has significant ongoing relationships with others (Nuffield Council on Bioethics, 2009).

Ethics of care in the memory clinic

Person-centred care (PCC), as discussed in Chapter 2, is an ethical approach to caring for persons living and dying with dementia, and evaluates the care being delivered as through the eyes of the person receiving that care (Adams, 2008). The team works in partnership with the patients and their family/carer to respect autonomy.

Assessment in the memory clinic

The clinic will undertake a comprehensive assessment using the approaches described previously in this chapter. This will occur in the clinic, but home visits are undertaken if necessary. As there is an emphasis on carer support, a detailed assessment of this is also undertaken. There is an assessment of educational needs for the person, their carer and their family so that appropriate information and education can be provided by the team. Although some assessments, such as a PET scan, are conducted just once, others, such as the MMSE and medication needs assessments, are ongoing.

> **Chapter summary**
>
> Assessing the care needs of a person who is confused and who may gain a diagnosis of dementia needs a comprehensive, multi-disciplinary approach. The nurse may undertake most of the assessment, but they also have a role in coordinating it. To undertake a comprehensive assessment, the nurse needs to explore the following elements: physiological; psychological; emotional; socio-cultural; environmental; spiritual.
>
> Specialist units such as memory clinics have the multi-disciplinary expertise to undertake this assessment. Some of these units are attached to physical adult services and some are attached to mental health services, but their assessment processes are similar.

Activities: brief outline answers

Activity 5.2: Critical thinking (page 82)

There are many reasons why Brenda may have been anxious and disorganised this Christmas. Brenda may have had a number of other unplanned things to do in the days coming up to Christmas; she may not have been able to get her shopping at the usual place or time. She may have had a late night or be feeling unwell.

Activity 5.3: Evidence-based practice and research (page 83)

There are a number of features you may have noted, including confusion, memory difficulties, repetition of words or sentences or requests, disorientation, anxiety and even aggression.

Activity 5.4: Critical thinking (page 86)

You were asked to consider how you would complete an assessment of Brenda. While undertaking your assessment you will also need to consider the significance of your findings. For example, you already know that Brenda had a temperature of 37.2°; this would be considered a low-grade pyrexia. On arrival in the ward you would need to repeat the observations. You may discover that Brenda's temperature is slightly higher. After her journey to hospital and stay in the accident and emergency department her temperature may have reduced. However, it is well known that infection can cause delirium. The sudden onset of confusion and agitation would also lead you to suspect delirium.

Activity 5.5: Critical thinking (page 89)

The advantages of an MRI or PET scan would allow the team to identify any structural changes in Brenda's brain and facilitate the diagnosis of dementia. A scan may find abnormalities that they were not looking for and not find the abnormalities they expected. Many people with dementia do not have structural changes, and others with structural changes do not have dementia. While MRIs and PET scans may help guide the diagnosis, they cannot give a definitive answer, and this can lead to increased anxiety in the person.

Activity 5.6: Critical thinking (page 93)

The gentleman 'wandering' up and down the corridor untying his pyjamas may be looking for a toilet or for his clothes to change into.

Activity 5.7: Communication (page 93)

As a nurse you need to demonstrate an attitude of respect for the person by actively listening to them and trying to understand what is happening to them. Do not respond in a negative way such as with embarrassment or horror. You should allow the person time to express their feelings, showing a relaxed and accepting or non-judgemental approach. You should promote a sense of safety and comfort.

Activity 5.8: Critical thinking (page 94)

The frequent changes of environment when admitted to hospital – the accident and emergency unit, the admissions unit, and then a ward that includes new staff – may increase Brenda's confusion and distress. If the lighting is kept on at night, she may not be aware of the time of day, and this may affect her ability to sleep. If Brenda does not get enough sleep, it will increase the confusion she is experiencing. Brenda may also be anxious about what is wrong with her and what the staff may need to do to her. Raised anxiety levels can create increased confusion.

Activity 5.9: Critical thinking (page 96)

The factors that may have influenced Brenda's low score on the MMSE are numerous and may include:

- anxiety;
- fear;
- lack of sleep;
- changes in her diet;
- infection;
- pain;
- noise;
- lighting.

Further reading

Neno, R, Aveyard, B and Heath, H (2007) *Older people and mental health nursing.* Oxford; Blackwell Publishing.

This book offers a concise overview of delirium in one chapter and depression in later life in another. Its language is easily accessed and well structured.

Useful websites

http://guidance.nice.org.uk/CG42

The National Institute for Health and Clinical Excellence website provides guidance on the use of the dementia care pathway it has developed, including the use of medication.

www.alzheimers.org.uk/site/scripts/documents_info.php?documentID=260

On the Alzheimer's Society website there is information on assessment that is not only useful for patients/carers but also for health care staff.

www.dh.gov.uk/health/2011/11/spotting-the-signs-of-dementia

Use this web link to find out more information about the Department of Health's campaign to raise awareness of the early signs and symptoms of dementia. Aimed at encouraging more people to seek an early diagnosis of dementia, the campaign targets the family and friends of people at risk of dementia who are likely to be the first to see the signs and can encourage their loved one to see their GP.

www.patient.co.uk/doctor/Screening-for-Cognitive-Impairment.htm

The Screening for cognitive impairment web page offers a number of psychological tests for cognitive impairment such as the GP COG, 6 CIT, IQ CODE, AMT and TYM test, all of which can help identify cognitive impairment.

www.stvincents.ie/dynamic/File/Addenbrookes_A_SVUH_MedEl_tool.pdf

This is a copy of the Addenbrooke's Cognitive Examination (ACE-R) screening tool used by many nurses and occupational therapists to assess dementia in the hospital situation. It takes some time and to attempt to complete it in one session can be difficult if the person has problems with attention or concentration as do most people with dementia.

Chapter 6
Diagnosis

NMC Standards for Pre-registration Nursing Education

This chapter will address issues within all four domains of the pre-registration nursing competencies but most significantly the following competencies:

Domain 1: Professional values

9. All nurses must appreciate the value of evidence in practice, be able to understand and appraise research, apply relevant theory and research findings to their work, and identify areas for further investigation.

Domain 3: Nursing practice and decision-making

7. All nurses must be able to recognise and interpret signs of normal and deteriorating mental and physical health and respond promptly to maintain or improve the health and comfort of the service user, acting to keep them and others safe.

NMC Essential Skills Clusters

This chapter will support the following ESCs:

Cluster: Care, compassion and communication

1. As partners in the care process, people can trust a newly registered graduate nurse to provide collaborative care based on the highest standards, knowledge and competence.

By entry to the register:

viii. Demonstrates clinical confidence through sound knowledge, skills and understanding relevant to field.

Cluster: Organisational aspects of care

16. People can trust the newly registered graduate nurse to safely lead, coordinate and manage care.

By entry to the register:

iii. Bases decisions on evidence and uses experience to guide decision-making.

> **Chapter aims**
>
> On completion of this chapter you should have developed an understanding of:
>
> - the common and differing features of the dementia subtypes;
> - the nurse's role in diagnosis;
> - sharing the diagnosis with the person and their family.

Introduction

A diagnosis of dementia gains different responses from each individual and their family. As you will read throughout this book, there is the need for us as nurses to see people as unique individuals who have different expectations and personal coping strategies. *The best thing for us was when he got the diagnosis and we had a title . . .we could say we know what it is* (Alzheimer's Society, 2008a, p28) was one response, and another was: *I might just as well kill myself then* (Alzheimer's Society, 2008a, p27). Terry Pratchett, the author, seeks to de-demonise the disease; he suggests:

> *The first step is to talk about dementia because it's a fact, well established in folklore, that if we are to kill the demon then first we have to say its name . . . Names have power like the word Alzheimer's; it terrorizes us. It has the power over us. When we are prepared to discuss it aloud we might have power over it. There should be no shame in having it yet people feel ashamed and people don't talk about it.*
> (Alzheimer's Society, 2008a, p8)

This chapter initially considers risk factors for dementia and definitions, and then goes on to explore each of the major subtypes of dementia in order of **prevalence**. It then discusses what are considered reversible dementias – HIV and alcohol dementia – and finally it explains the nurse's role when giving the diagnosis.

Risk factors for developing dementia

Many people are worried about developing dementia, given that there is no cure for this degenerative disease. While there is no vaccination or inoculation available, it is worth recognising the risk factors associated with its development. Many of these we have no control over as individuals, but there are ways we can improve or maintain our health to reduce the risk of developing diseases such as dementia.

> **Activity 6.1**   *Critical thinking*
>
> Spend a few minutes thinking about how you could improve or maintain your health and reduce your chances of becoming unwell.
>
> *There is an outline answer at the end of the chapter.*

Activity 6.1 asked you to consider how you might improve or maintain your health. As nurses, it is important that we understand how to do this both for our clients and for ourselves. Some of the health promotion activities you identified you might not have thought were relevant to dementia, but look at the risk factors described by the authors in Table 6.1 and see whether you think that some of the general healthy living advice is relevant to dementia.

As you can see in Table 6.1, there are a number of risk factors that you will have no control over, but there are some where following healthy living advice can reduce your risk. All of the authors identify the risks of age, gender and genetics, which at the moment there is no cure for. There are, though, many factors in the list that you may have control over.

- Trauma by reducing risk-taking behaviour.
- Toxicity by reducing alcohol consumption and smoking.
- Transmittable diseases by infection control and safe sex.
- Other diseases such as cardiovascular disorders by healthy lifestyles.

These approaches will reduce your risk, but even if you follow all the healthy living guidance, you may still develop dementia; there is a lot we do not know about this disease.

Cantley (2001)	Cox and Keady (1999)	Cheston and Bender (1999)	Alzheimer's Society (2010b)
		Increasing age	
Degenerative disorders such as multiple sclerosis, cardiovascular disease, Parkinson's; genetic disorders such as Down's syndrome and Huntingdon's chorea			
Traumatic; head injury			
Transmissible: AIDS, CJD, syphilis	Infections		HIV/AIDS
Toxic: such as alcohol, CO_2, trace elements, smoking			
Space-occupying lesions			
Metabolic such as hypothyroidism, diabetes, oestrogen deficiency			
	Lack of vitamins	Education and occupation – poor education is linked with poor health choices (diet/exercise etc.)	Lifestyle choices
		Depression	

Table 6.1: Risk factors for developing dementia

Defining dementia

The National Dementia Strategy *Living well with dementia* (DH, 2009) defines dementia as a **syndrome** that:

> *may be caused by a number of illnesses in which there is progressive decline in multiple areas of function, including decline in memory, reasoning, communication skills and the ability to carry out daily activities. Alongside this decline, individuals may develop behavioural and psychological symptoms such as depression, psychosis, aggression and wandering.*

Two diagnostic tools used in the UK to make medical diagnoses of brain diseases are *The international classification of disease* (ICD), version 10, and *Diagnostic statistical manual* (DSM), version 4 (IV). The ICD-10 has recently been updated (2010) and the DSM-V is expected to be available in 2013, but given changes in psychiatry, the DSM-IV was updated in 2000; this edition is referred to as the DSM text revision IV (DSM-IV-TR). The diagnostic criteria for mental health problems have changed over the years, which is why these diagnostic tools are frequently updated. In the past the diagnostic criteria for each system were quite different, but the current versions are more similar, although they still have differences.

ICD defines dementia as:

> *a syndrome due to disease of the brain, usually of a chronic or progressive nature, in which there is disturbance of **multiple higher cortical functions**, including memory, thinking, orientation, comprehension, calculation, learning capacity, language, and judgement. Consciousness is not clouded. The impairments of cognitive function are commonly accompanied, and occasionally preceded, by deterioration in emotional control, social behaviour, or motivation.*
> (WHO, 2010)

DSM-IV-TR (APA, 2011) defines dementia as *significant impairment of the person's memory for new and previously learnt information*. One or more of the following must also be present.

- **Dysphasia/aphasia** – difficulty with the use of verbal language or absence of language. This can be seen in the loss of proper nouns, echoing what other people say, repetition of words or phrases.
- **Apraxia** – loss of the ability to undertake intentional movement, such as being able to tie shoe laces.
- **Agnosia** – loss of the ability to recognise objects; the person may even lack recognition of members of their family.
- **Impaired higher cortical functioning** – lack of the ability to undertake abstract thinking or complex behaviours such as planning a trip or cooking a meal.

According to the DSM-IC-TR, the disturbances in the specific criteria should be severe enough to cause problems in the person's life and must show deterioration from previous functioning. In addition to the changes in cognitive functioning indicated above, the symptoms of dementia may also include personality changes and a lack of emotional stability.

The definitions of dementia given above appear to be very similar, but the definition given in the National Dementia Strategy is in the most accessible language, probably due to the intended readership – the public rather than health care professionals. Dementia is a diagnosis by exclusion: in order to diagnose dementia, other disorders that can cause similar symptoms need first to be excluded.

Common features of dementia

The definitions and diagnostic criteria offered above provide us with the signs that we, as nurses, need to aware of in our caring roles. The common features are:

*   loss of memory;
*   difficulty in finding the right words or understanding what people are saying;
*   difficulty in performing previously routine tasks;
*   personality and mood changes.
    (ADI, 2011)

How these signs are observed in people will not only be influenced by the type of dementia they have, but also vary quite dramatically in how they are experienced by the individual person.

Activity 6.3   *Critical thinking*

Reconsider your responses to Activity 6.1. Are the signs you identified the same as those provided above by Alzheimer's Disease International? In what ways do they differ?

As this is based on a personal response, there is no outline answer at the end of the chapter.

Diagnostic assessment for suspected dementia

As a nurse, you will recognise that the common features of dementia could be due to many other factors. In Chapter 5 we considered the **differential diagnosis** of delirium, and through case studies in previous chapters we have discovered that problems such as stress and infections could also give rise to these features. When doctors or nurse specialists assess an individual presenting with the symptoms of dementia, therefore, they need to undertake a comprehensive assessment, including a detailed health and social history.

The Department of Health (2011b) issued guidance on the assessment and diagnosis of dementia (*Service specification for dementia: memory service for early diagnosis and intervention*), emphasising the importance of a broad and comprehensive assessment. Ideally, the patient's next of kin (NOK) should be involved, to provide information on the impact of the disease on the individual, and themselves. The significance of early diagnosis is clear, since you would want the patient to be able to say who their NOK is, and how much they want their NOK involved, while they still have the capacity. The diagnosis of a dementia is said to be one given not only to the patient but to their NOK as well. As the disease progresses, its impact on the NOK increases as they inevitably have to take on more responsibility in the care of the patient. Early diagnosis helps the NOK prepare for the next stage.

History taking

Nursing assessment and history taking were considered in Chapter 5, but it is important to briefly revisit it here. History taking includes, but is not limited to:

- a subjective and objective assessment of the patient's life, social, family and carer history, circumstances and preferences, as well as their physical and mental health needs and current level of functioning and abilities, including an interview with an informant (usually carer/family) to generate a collateral history;
- assessment of history and impacts of impairments of vision, hearing and mobility;
- assessment of history and impacts of impairments of medical co-morbidities;
- assessment of key psychiatric and behavioural features, including depression, wandering and psychosis;
- risk assessment covering all areas appropriate to the individual, e.g. falls, risk to self, child care or carer responsibilities, driving and financial and legal issues;
- carer assessment, including burden, health and function.
  (DH, 2011b)

As well as history taking, the health care provider should note who the person wishes to be informed of the diagnosis, the process and time lines (NICE/SCIE, 2006).

The person should receive a comprehensive neurological examination along with an exploration of their health history. They should also have a number of blood tests including:

- complete blood count;
- electrolytes;
- calcium;
- glucose;
- blood urea;
- nitrogen/creatinine;
- liver function tests;
- thyroid function tests;
- serum B12 level;
- syphilis serology.

Depending on the person's history, other blood tests such as serum folate, HIV testing and a toxicology screen or a lumbar puncture may be necessary. Taking X-ray pictures and urinalysis are also important. If an alternative explanation for the features common to dementia have not been established at this stage, neuro-imaging such as CAT or MRI scans along with neuro-psychological testing will be undertaken (some of these were discussed in Chapter 5). Even after all these tests misdiagnosis occurs, and a definite subtype cannot be confirmed until after a post-mortem examination (Brunnstrom et al., 2009).

Despite the complexity and skill required with obtaining a diagnosis, the government emphasises the need for early diagnosis to provide appropriate and early intervention to ensure the best quality of life for the person with dementia (DH, 2009).

The Department of Health (2011b) recommends the pathway shown in Figure 6.1 when a diagnosis of dementia is made.

There are many types of dementia, but the most common in those over the age of 65 years is Alzheimer's disease (62 per cent). In those with early onset dementia (younger than 65 years) 34 per cent have Alzheimer's. This indicates that 66 per cent of those suffering early onset dementia are likely to have symptoms that are modifiable – hence the need for accurate diagnosis (Harvey et al., 2003). As Alzheimer's is the most prevalent type of dementia, it will be considered first.

Alzheimer's dementia

Alzheimer's dementia was first described in 1906 by Alois Alzheimer, after whom it is named. Initially, it was used to identify early onset (before 65) dementia, as cognitive impairment after

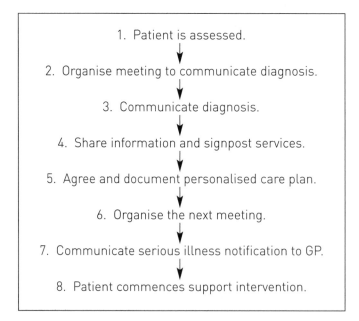

Figure 6.1: Dementia care pathway

this time was wrongly considered to be part of normal ageing. More recently, the term Alzheimer's dementia has been used as an umbrella term for most types of dementia, but in health care we differentiate between dementias using the diagnostic tools mentioned above.

The disease process that Alzheimer identified involves the destruction of brain cells in areas of the brain responsible for memory. This affects the person's ability to remember, think and make decisions. It is not known what causes this condition, although there are some biological theories.

The diagnostic criteria for Alzheimer's dementia can be found in Part 5 (mental and behavioural disorders) of the ICD-10. For late onset Alzheimer's, the primary feature is slow progressive memory loss, but early onset dementia involves deterioration in wider higher cortical functioning. The main criteria for diagnosis is an insidious progression of degenerative cerebral disease with **neuropathological** and **neurochemical** features.

Neuropathological features

Shrinkage, including reduction of fluid gaps, develops in the **temporal lobe** and **hippocampus**, which are responsible for storing and retrieving new information.

Senile plaques are made of clusters of insoluble fibrils consisting of beta amyloid protein. These plaques surround nerve cells and kill them. They also trigger an inflammatory response, which releases more beta amyloid protein leading to chronic brain inflammation and more plaques.

Neurofibrillary tangles (NFT) develop from within the neurone. Another protein, tau, has been implicated in this and interferes with the normal functioning of the neurone.

Neurochemical features

Acetylcholine (ACh), a neurotransmitter, is reduced by 60 per cent or more in the **cerebral cortex** in Alzheimer's disease.

An excessive amount of glutamate, another neurotransmitter, is found in the brain in Alzheimer's disease.

Symptom profile of a person with Alzheimer's dementia

This can initially include:

*   lapses of memory;
*   difficulty in finding the right words for everyday objects;
*   mood swings.

This can lead on to:

*   forgetting recent events, names, faces;
*   difficulty with language;
*   confusion with money or driving a car (getting lost on familiar routes);
*   mood swings involving being tearful for no apparent reason or thinking someone is going to hurt them.

In the later stages people may also:

- behave in what is considered bizarre ways, such as wandering at night, or being inappropriately dressed;
- lose their inhibitions and sense of suitable behaviour for the situation.
(Alzheimer's Society, 2010b)

Reread the case study of Brenda Drake in Chapter 5 to help your understanding of Alzheimer's dementia.

Vascular dementia

Vascular dementia is the second most prevalent type in those aged over 65 years, with 27 per cent of those diagnosed being placed in this category or mixed Alzheimer's and vascular dementia (Alzheimer's Society, 2011). It is estimated that about 18 per cent of those under 65 with dementia have vascular dementia, which makes its prevalence similar to other non-Alzheimer's dementias in this age group (Harvey et al., 2003). Vascular dementia is described as having a '**stepwise**' progression: a person suddenly deteriorates and then remains stable for a while and then takes another 'step' down in ability. These steps may be quite focal, so specific skills are lost and others remain; for example, there could be a loss of language skills but memory and reasoning remain intact.

Our brains, as with other organs, need a good supply of blood to maintain health and function properly. Blood is supplied to the brain by the circulatory system: the cardio (heart) vascular (blood vessels: arteries, capillaries, etc.) system. When our cardiovascular system is not working effectively, the blood does not reach all the areas of our body and cells die. If the blood does not get to the brain cells and they die, this can lead to a condition known as a cerebral-vascular accident (CVA or stroke) and the onset of vascular dementia.

There are a number of health problems that can cause vascular dementia, including high blood pressure, heart problems, high blood cholesterol and diabetes. These conditions also put the person at risk of a stroke, which can affect other areas of the body as well as brain function. There are many different types of vascular dementia but the two main types are caused by stroke, and frequently referred to as **multi-infarct** dementia and small vessel disease: these can also occur together.

Multi-infarct dementia occurs when there is sudden loss of blood to an area of the brain usually due to obstruction but also by bleeding. This type of vascular dementia is known as a **cortical encephalopathy** (a disease of the outer part of the brain).

Small vessel disease is a **sub-cortical encephalopathy** (a disease of the inner part of the brain). It is usually more insidious in nature, and a severe form is Binswanger's disease. It is caused by damage to the tiny blood vessels deep within the brain. It occurs when these small blood vessels 'fur up' and block the blood supply. The symptoms for this type of vascular dementia are often accompanied by walking problems (Alzheimer's Society, 2011).

Symptom profile in vascular dementia

The symptoms that can occur with vascular dementia are very diverse and depend on where the blood supply was interrupted. As already identified, the progression can also be quite varied due to the cause and treatment received.

However, a person with vascular dementia will have a symptom profile that differs from other dementias in a number of ways. People with vascular dementia may particularly experience:

- a 'stepped' progression;
- concentration and communication problems;
- depression;
- symptoms associated with stroke such as muscle weakness;
- memory problems, but this is not necessarily a primary feature as it is for Alzheimer's;
- epilepsy;
- acute confusion.

Other symptoms may include:

- misperception;
- wandering and getting lost;
- restlessness;
- incontinence.

As nurses, we need to remember to consider the whole person, as can be seen in the case study of Mary in Chapter 1. Mental health, psychological well-being and physical health are intrinsically linked. Activities undertaken to improve physical health, such as exercise and healthy eating, are just as necessary for mental and psychological well-being.

Dementia with Lewy bodies

Dementia with Lewy bodies (DLB) has features of both Alzheimer's dementia and Parkinson's disease, and about 10 per cent of people of all ages diagnosed with dementia are in this category. Alzheimer's dementia was described earlier in this chapter due to its high prevalence rate; Parkinson's disease will be briefly outlined here.

Parkinson's disease is a progressive neurological condition that is experienced by one person in every 500 in the UK (120,000 people). One in 20 people with Parkinson's is between the age of 20 and 40, but most are over 50. In Parkinson's disease there is death of the brain cells that produce dopamine, a neurotransmitter, in an area known as the substantia nigra deep in the brain. Symptoms are usually divided into motor and non-motor. The motor symptoms are tremor, rigidity and slowness. Non-motor symptoms include pain, depression, sweating and constipation. Lewy bodies are also found in people experiencing this condition, and many of them go on to develop dementia that resembles DLB.

What are Lewy bodies?

Lewy bodies are tiny spherical protein deposits found in brain cells; they are named after the doctor who identified them in 1912. These deposits interrupt the chemical messengers in the brain called neurotransmitters, particularly acetylcholine (ACh) and dopamine. As we saw earlier, ACh was implicated in the symptoms of Alzheimer's dementia, and lack of dopamine is the key cause of Parkinson's disease. It is unclear how Lewy bodies affect the functioning of these two neurotransmitters, but there is evidence to support this theory.

Symptom profile of Lewy body dementia

As with Alzheimer's dementia, DLB is a progressive degenerative disease and so symptoms become worse over time. The symptoms experienced are similar to those of Alzheimer's dementia and Parkinson's disease, and include:

- problems with attention, alertness, disorientation;
- higher cortical functions such as planning and problem solving;
- memory problems, which are usually less severe than in Alzheimer's dementia;
- muscle stiffness and trembling of limbs;
- shuffling gait;
- loss of facial expression;
- changes in voice.

They may also experience:

- detailed hallucinations;
- rapid variations in ability;
- falling asleep during the day but disturbed nights;
- fainting, falling, 'funny turns'.
  (Alzheimer's Society, 2011)

Read the case study of Neil Brown to gain further insight into this disorder.

Case study: Neil Brown

Neil is a 44-year-old man with a wife, Tessa, and two children who are 10 and 14 years old. Neil's wife happily tells people that Neil's cup was always half empty whereas hers was always half full, but between them they probably had a balanced view of the world. They were married quite young but waited for a while to have children as Neil needed to make sure the time was right. They were a close family and needed few other friends. A couple of years ago Tessa became concerned about Neil as his mood had appeared to become low and his anxiety increased; he also seemed to have a fine tremor. She encouraged him to see the GP, who like Tessa thought Neil was anxious and depressed. The GP tried to encourage Neil to accept some counselling through the 'Improving access to psychological therapy' service, but he was unhappy about doing this. The GP referred him to the local Community Mental Health Team for further assessment. Neil was assessed by the psychiatrist for anxiety and depression, but he did not appear to fulfil the criteria for moderate depression or anxiety. There were

continued . . .

signs such as low mood, slowness of movement, poor attention and memory problems, but the psychiatrist felt that a differential diagnosis of Parkinson's disease could also be made, so Neil was referred to a neurologist.

Neil was happy to see the neurologist, and his wife went with him as her concern was rising. The neurologist took an extensive history and conducted some neurological tests. A diagnosis of Parkinson's is made on the basis of 'clinical judgement' as there is no definitive test. The neurologist did not feel there was enough evidence to provide a diagnosis of Parkinson's, so they sent Neil for an MRI scan. Parkinson's cannot be detected on an MRI but other changes can. The neurologist's report and the MRI report were sent to the GP, who referred Neil back to the psychiatrist. Based on the initial psychiatric report, the neurologist's report and the MRI scan, Neil was reassessed, and it was decided that the most probable diagnosis for Neil was Lewy body dementia.

Activity 6.4   *Critical thinking*

How do you think a diagnosis of Lewy body dementia might affect Neil's life?

An outline answer is given at the end of the chapter.

A diagnosis of dementia can be problematic at any age but for younger people, like Neil, who have employment, children and mortgages to consider, it can be even more difficult to gain a sense of well-being. Nurses can guide people like him to access the available support services.

Fronto-temporal lobar degeneration (FTLD)

This term is used for a number of conditions, including Pick's disease and dementia associated with motor neurone disease. Despite being quite rare, it is the second or third most common early onset dementia (Alzheimer's Society, 2010b). FTLD is recognised as representing only 8 per cent of the total number of people with dementia, but in the early onset group it accounts for the same number of people as those with vascular dementia (18 per cent) (Harvey et al., 2003). All of these dementias are caused by damage to the frontal lobe and/or temporal lobe of the brain. FTLD has three types: fronto-temporal dementia (FTD) (changes in behaviour/personality and executive function; deterioration in problem solving ability); semantic dementia (lack of semantics or meaning and understanding); and non-fluent aphasia (significant deterioration of speech). The different labels refer to the symptoms observed.

Symptom profile of a person with FTLD

The symptom profile of a person with FTLD is quite wide and will involve behavioural/personality changes, executive function problems, understanding and speech. A person with FTLD tends to have changes in their eating patterns, although the first signs of the disorder are usually behaviours that seem out of character. The variations in personality and behaviour may include:

- loss of inhibitions or increased extroversion;
- spending money excessively;
- apathy or withdrawal from social activities;
- loss of empathy;
- changes in sexual behaviour;
- becoming distractible;
- development of fixed routines or becoming obsessive;
- development of a sweet tooth and/or overeating, leading to weight gain;
- decreased amount of speech or repetitive speech;
- lack of insight.

The FTLD subtype fronto-temporal dementia (FTD) divides further into frontal lobe degeneration type, Pick type and motor neurone type. In frontal lobe degeneration you will primarily see changes in behaviour and/or personality and executive functioning, whereas Pick's is also associated with speech difficulties. Pick's dementia can be diagnosed on MRI scans by the large protein tangles that are called Pick bodies after the professor of psychiatry who identified them.

The clinical picture of FTD with motor neurone disease differs from Pick's in that the personality disintegrates less and personal contact is preserved. The age of onset is between 38 and 78 and on average 55, with the **mean** (type of average) age of death in the late fifties. As with other types of FTD, the main initial changes are uninhibited behaviour and personality changes. Other significant changes are:

- deficits in memory;
- intellectual impairment;
- emotional problems;
- deficits in speech production.

Apraxia (loss of ability of movement) and agnosia (loss of recognition), seen in Alzheimer's, are not usually present in this disorder. These symptoms tend to occur prior to any of the motor neurone disease (MND) symptoms, which occur about six to 12 months afterwards (Mitsuyama and Inoue, 2009). Read the case study of Maeve to further develop your insight into FTD with MND.

Case study: Maeve O'Rourke

Maeve is 50 years old and lived with her partner in a quiet suburb of a large city. She worked as a solicitor and has always been considered to be professional in all her work activities. Over a couple of months Maeve became more irritable with people at work and made a few mistakes, but, given her age, most people, including her partner, thought this was due to the menopause. Maeve's behaviour continued to deteriorate and she started to 'flirt' with some of the young men and invite them to her house, saying her husband would not be in. She then attempted to sit on a client's knee, at which point she was suspended from work. Because of her partner's insistence, she went to see her GP, and her GP requested an urgent psychiatric assessment. On assessment, no

continued . . .

signs of psychosis were detected – no delusions or hallucinations. It was therefore not possible to detain her in a psychiatric hospital when she refused to be admitted voluntarily. The psychiatrist suspected alcohol or drug misuse, but there was no evidence to support this. Maeve agreed to attend the general hospital for an MRI scan. On the scan, atrophy in the fronto-temporal lobe was observed. Maeve's behaviour continued to deteriorate and her speech became slurred; she was irritable and aggressive towards her husband and sexually disinhibited in public. Eventually, a member of the public contacted the police, who believed she was mentally ill and escorted her to the psychiatric hospital under section 136 of the Mental Health Act. At the hospital this was converted to section 2 of the Mental Health Act so that she could be assessed over a period of 28 days. During this period Maeve started to have problems with moving around and her muscles started to twitch. With the results of the MRI and her psychiatric assessment, she was diagnosed with fronto-temporal dementia with motor neurone disease. Given Maeve's lack of insight into her condition, residential care was sought for her despite her age.

The case study of Maeve demonstrates how problematic diagnosis is and how the earlier an accurate diagnosis can be given the higher the likelihood of appropriate treatment and maintenance of quality of life. If Maeve, with encouragement from her family, had had her symptoms investigated earlier instead of assuming they were due to the menopause, some of the distress experienced by her and those in contact with her might have been ameliorated. She might also have had the opportunity to plan for her future.

Activity 6.5   *Critical thinking*

If you had met Maeve before hearing her diagnosis, how do you think you would have interpreted her behaviour?

As this is a personal reflection, there is no outline answer at the end of the chapter.

Alzheimer's, vascular, dementia with Lewy bodies and fronto-temporal dementia are the most common types of dementia, and all have neuropathological and neurochemical changes. The following dementias are rarer and are primarily due to infection or toxicity.

Creutzfeldt-Jakob disease

Creutzfeldt-Jakob disease (CJD) is a prion disease; it is very rare and accounts for only 0.1 per cent of people who have dementia. A prion is a misfolded protein that is infectious; when it enters the body of animals, including humans, it induces other proteins to misfold as well. These develop into **fibrils** (fine fibres) that knit together to create mats and holes like a sponge, hence the term 'spongiform' used in the medical term for CJD: transmissible spongiform encephalopathy.

Prions can occur in the brain for a number of years before any symptoms are shown, but when they do, progression of the disease is rapid. Progression is usually measured in months rather than years.

There are fours types of CJD.

- **Sporadic** – occurs without an identified cause usually in people over 50.
- **Iatrogenic** – occurs because of medical treatment such as a corneal transplant.
- **Familial** – genetic disorder usually occurring between the ages of 20 and 60.
- **Variant** – caused by eating infected foods; average age of death is 29.

Symptom profile of CJD

Early symptoms are:

- lapses of memory;
- mood changes;
- apathy;
- clumsiness;
- confusion;
- unsteady gait;
- slow slurred speech.

Later symptoms are:

- jerky movements;
- stiffness;
- incontinence;
- immobility;
- aphasia.

Read the case study of Karen to develop your understanding of this disorder and consider the nursing care she might need.

Case study: Karen Best

Karen is 18 years old and working on her A levels. She had always been a conscientious student and did well in her GCSEs; she hoped to become a vet. Karen's parents became worried about her when she started to lose interest in her studies and her friends. They were afraid she was becoming stressed and exhausted due to studying and having a part-time job in the local supermarket. They encouraged Karen to resign from her job to allow her to study. Despite the reduction in work, Karen showed less interest in her studies and spent a lot of time on her bed not interacting. Karen's mother took her to the GP, who suggested that she should speak to the counsellor attached to her school as Karen said she would feel comfortable talking to them. Over the next few weeks Karen's mood appeared to swing from being quietly tearful to being irritable and argumentative. At this stage Karen shared some of her thoughts with the school counsellor, who was concerned that Karen might be experiencing some psychotic symptoms and therefore contacted her parents, recommending that she was taken to see her GP urgently. The GP was able to refer Karen to the early interventions in psychosis team, who undertook a comprehensive assessment with her.

continued . . . •••

Karen asked for her mother to be present during the assessment. During the assessment it became apparent that although Karen had mood swings, some delusional thoughts and hallucinations, she also had some slurred speech and appeared unsteady on her feet. The team established that Karen did not use alcohol or any other drugs, so they felt she needed to be referred to a neurologist. By the time Karen had seen the neurologist her symptoms had progressed significantly, she was now struggling with speech and walking, and showed some signs of confusion. An urgent MRI was conducted, and it was established that Karen probably had a form of CJD – most likely the variant type. Karen was nursed at home by her parents with the support of the paediatric palliative care team until she died ten months after showing signs of the disease.

Due to the usually rapid disease process of CJD, as seen in the case study of Karen, it could be argued that it does not fully comply with the definition of dementia, but it is generally recognised as such. The last two types of dementia that are going to be considered here are more disputably labelled dementia, particularly alcohol-induced, because they are reversible.

Human immunodeficiency virus (HIV) related dementia

In the 1980s there was a huge public awareness campaign related to HIV (human immuno-deficiency virus) and AIDS (acquired immune deficiency syndrome). This identified how the infection could be caught and the high risk of early death. People were advised not to share needles and to practise 'safe sex'. Nurses saw the introduction of increased infection control polices to reduce the risk of contamination through infected body fluids. In those early public health campaigns there was no mention of the risk of early onset dementia.

Dementia associated with HIV has become one the most feared aspects of the progression of this viral infection. It has had many labels, such as AIDS dementia complex, HIV dementia and HIV encephalopathy. It has decreased since the introduction of antiretroviral medication. The Alzheimer's Society (2010b) stated that 40 per cent of those with HIV were expected to develop dementia, but since the introduction of antiretroviral therapy (HAART) the percentage has been about 20 (a 50 per cent reduction). Nath et al. (2008) agree that the rate of HIV dementia has changed with the introduction of HAART, but their figures show a 15–50 per cent reduction, and Jamieson (1999) states that 90 per cent of those dying of AIDS have signs of brain damage at the post-mortem examination. Nath et al. (2008) go on to say that, despite HAART, there are more people with HIV dementia. This is due to people living longer with HIV, as HAART has reduced early mortality caused by other conditions. There are four types of HIV dementia.

1. *Subacute progressive* – dementia is progressing because the HIV is not being treated.
2. *Chronic active* – associated with poor adherence to HAART or limited therapeutic effect, so HIV is still active but progression of dementia is slowed.
3. *Chronic inactive* – there is good adherence to HAART and effective viral suppression; HIV is still present but progression of dementia has been stopped.

4. *Reversible* – the symptoms of dementia have diminished due to good adherence to HAART and effective suppression.

Life expectancy for those experiencing HIV dementia in groups 1 and 2 is between six months and two years (Nath et al., 2008).

Symptom profile of HIV dementia

Nath et al. (2008) state that symptoms in the early stages include:

- short-term memory loss;
- executive function reduced, reasoning etc.;
- mental and physical slowing;
- reading and comprehension difficulties;
- apathy;
- walking problems – gait, stumbling;
- postural tremor.

Jamieson (1999) identifies a small subset of people experiencing HIV dementia as having symptoms that include mania, psychoses and bizarre behaviour. He states that as the disease progresses problems with concentration, reading, writing and language occur.

In the later stages, Nath et al. (2008) describe:

- widespread difficulties;
- **myelopathy** (damage to spinal cord) and **neuropathy** (damage to nerves);
- impairment of everyday functioning.

The symptoms listed by the Alzheimer's Society (2010b) include those identified by both Jamieson (1999) and Nath et al. (2008) but without the recognition of sub-groups and stages.

The case study of Naomi indicates how the very young may be affected by this condition.

Case study: Naomi Polanski

Naomi was born in Moldavia and was brought by her parents to the UK when she was five years old. Naomi's parents registered with a GP in the UK and the health visitor (HV) assessed her development. The HV was a little concerned as Naomi appeared underweight and lethargic. The HV arranged to visit the family at home to see if she could gauge what was happening. On the home visit they found Naomi's mother in tears because Naomi was less responsive than she had been. According to the mother, Naomi had been a bright chatty child before they had moved to the UK. The HV rang the GP and it was organised for Naomi and her mother to be admitted to the children's ward so that Naomi could be thoroughly assessed. On admission, a number of tests were carried out, including blood tests. The blood tests showed that Naomi was HIV positive. Her mother and father were encouraged to be tested as well and it was found that her mother was also HIV positive. Both mother and child were commenced on antiretroviral therapy. Initially, Naomi appeared to respond well to the therapy – she moved around more easily and smiled at people – but her language skills did not return.

Dementia can affect any age group, but it is very rare in young people. The evidence available for HIV dementia has been developed in the USA, UK and Europe, where the strain of HIV is slightly different from that in Africa, which has the greatest prevalence rate. Africa also has the least access to antiretroviral therapy. We may therefore see large numbers of young people with HIV dementia in this area in the future.

Korsakoff's/alcohol dementia

Although older people have problems with alcohol dependency, alcohol-related dementia is a significant area of concern for those under 65; it accounts for 10 per cent of dementia experienced by this group (Harvey et al., 2003). It does, though, have one of the best prognoses – the highest chance of being reversible.

Korsakoff's dementia has been known by a number of labels: Korsakoff's amnesiac syndrome, Korsakoff's psychosis, alcohol dementia. There has been a lot of discussion about whether Korsakoff's dementia exists, and Korsakoff's psychosis has been dismissed. It was thought to be a psychosis due to the strong acceptance of **confabulated** stories by the person experiencing this problem, but these are no longer considered delusions. There is, though, agreement that alcohol can cause brain damage. Korsakoff's has been linked with Wernicke's encephalopathy: Wernicke-Korsakoff syndrome (WKS). Wernicke's encephalopathy is an acute neurological illness whereas Korsakoff's amnesiac or dementia is a chronic psychiatric disorder.

These conditions are related to a thiamine (vitamin B1) deficiency but some people with alcohol dementia do not have this vitamin deficiency and the damage is identified as due to the toxic effect of alcohol itself (Crowe, 1999). When people drink alcohol to excess they may become malnourished as alcohol reduces the body's ability to process nutrients and frequently people who drink excessive alcohol do not eat a balanced diet.

Symptom profile of the two components of WKS

According to the Alzheimer's Society (Alzheimer's Society, 2010b), the main symptoms of Wernicke's are:

- jerky movements or paralysis of the eye (eye problems);
- problems with balance and walking (ataxia);
- sleepiness and confusion (acute confusion).

In the case of Korsakoff's dementia people suffer from:

- problems with learning new information and skills – but normal short-term memory;
- lack of insight;
- personality changes;
- **confabulation** – filling gaps in memory with stories that may be extremely fanciful.

The most important part of nursing care is to encourage the person to abstain from drinking alcohol so that the damage is minimised. Both of these sets of problems are treated with vitamin supplements and this treatment is very effective – although if left untreated, Wernicke's can lead to death. Vitamin supplements usually facilitate a return to more normal functioning, but there is no evidence to suggest that they can undo the brain damage (Nath et al., 2008).

As you can see, labelling Korsakoff's as a dementia is problematic because if the person abstains from drinking alcohol and takes vitamin supplements, their condition may not feature *chronic progressive decline*.

Alcohol dementia without WKS usually presents itself in a similar manner to FTD dementia. The presenting features are dependent on where the damage occurs, but as with WKS there is the possibility of full remission if the person abstains from alcohol use (Crowe, 1999).

Read the case study of Mike to develop your understanding of how a person might experience alcohol dementia.

Case study: Mike

Over the years Mike had managed to reduce his drinking and at times stopped, but when things got too difficult for him he again returned to drinking. His wife continued to love and care for him with support from his care coordinator and the Alcoholics Anonymous family support group. When intoxicated, Mike became irritable and morose, but he was never aggressive to his wife or children. His drinking did cause some financial problems, but as a family they managed this.

When Mike reached the age of 50, Anita started to become concerned about him. He started returning late home from work but did not smell of alcohol. If she asked him where he had been, he gave rather long and difficult-to-believe stories of how he had been delayed. She also found him occasionally standing in the middle of the room looking distant. A couple of times when she asked what was wrong he snapped at her that nothing was wrong, which was out of character for him. Mike's drinking appeared to be reducing, and initially she put the changes down to this, but she was concerned that he had found another woman.

Anita was anxious, so she asked Mike if she could meet with his care coordinator with him to discuss her concerns. He was happy with this and explained to them both that there was no other woman, but he gave a rather long, detailed explanation about his moments of absence and coming home late. His care coordinator knew him well and recognised there was a problem, so they organised further assessments. These assessments indicated that Mike was suffering from alcohol dementia.

So far Mike's wife and children had provided most of his support. His care coordinator has offered long-term support with his problems and the mental health addictions service has provided treatment for him. The family had gained support from Alcoholics Anonymous family support (Al-Anon). Mike was given advice and support to stop drinking alcohol altogether, but two years later he was still having memory problems, was at times irritable with his family and a number of times returned home in a dishevelled state, giving explanations that his family found difficult to believe. Mike's place of work had tried to be supportive, but his behaviour led to two written warnings and he is very likely to lose his job.

Activity 6.6   *Critical thinking*

Read the case study of Mike. Given the brain damage caused by alcohol use, what sort of support do you think he and his family will need? Who will provide this support?

An outline answer is provided at the end of the chapter.

In Mike's case study you can see that most of his long-term support was provided by his family, his care coordinator (a nurse) and Al-Anon. Given his age, he will need additional support, as he is in paid employment, which will be paying for rent or mortgage, gas, electricity, etc. and he has a young family. He will need to negotiate and make plans for how he will manage if and when his condition deteriorates. The nurse and his family will need to offer him support and encouragement to facilitate his achievement of this.

The nurse's role in diagnosis

Nurses are integral to the diagnostic process; some specialist nurses undertake the diagnosis, but nurses are involved in every step even if a doctor is making the diagnosis. The nurse's contribution is invaluable in the comprehensive assessment required of the degree and effect of the symptoms of dementia on the individual. Whichever field of nursing you work in, you could be involved in the diagnosis of dementia, which affects one in four hospital in-patients (Alzheimer's Society, 2009). As nurses, we develop close relationships with people and their families, and it is through these that an accurate diagnosis can be made. Diagnosis of dementia is not clear-cut; it is easy to make a misdiagnosis, which could have huge implications for the person. You need to listen carefully to the person and their family in order not to miss that vital information. We need to be mindful of differential diagnosis – for example, if the person is more likely to have delirium or depression (see Chapter 5) or if the person has a reversible dementia such as alcohol-induced dementia.

Nurses undertake psychometric testing and collect observed information, but the most important role they fulfil is to emotionally support the person and their family, explaining to them what is happening and listening to their concerns.

Sharing the diagnosis

The *Dementia: out of the shadows* report commissioned by the Alzheimer's Society (2008a) clearly states that the diagnosis of dementia is a complex undertaking. Despite this, a diagnosis is important because it allows the person and their family the opportunity to adjust, make plans and consider treatment and care options.

If a psychiatrist or gerontologist has made the diagnosis of dementia, it is likely they will have shared this with the person and their family with a nurse in attendance. The nurse will then be able to spend time with the person and their family checking their understanding and current needs. The *Dementia: out of the shadows* report (Alzheimer's Society, 2008a) identifies how traumatic the experience of being given a diagnosis of dementia can be: Terry Pratchett, the author, likened it to being on the brink of hell. It also highlights some issues that we as nurses need to take into consideration when supporting people at this time.

People want to be taken seriously and listened to, so we need to ensure that we demonstrate good communication skills, giving accurate information in a jargon-free language that can be understood. The family's views and concerns need to be respected alongside those of the person with dementia. Referrals need to be made sensitively and swiftly: being responded to in a positive manner helps people to cope with the situation (Alzheimer's Society, 2008a). Using the humanised person-centred approach, focusing on the person's strengths rather than focusing on what they cannot do, will facilitate a greater sense of well-being. One person in the *Dementia: out of the shadows* report said: *If anything was destined to make you feel better it was the actual attention they gave you* (Alzheimer's Society, 2008a, p26).

We need to respect and value people's abilities and give them time and attention. We need to humanise our care to ensure people with dementia gain quality of life and a sense of well-being. The Nuffield Council of Bioethics has produced recommendations when considering the ethical issues surrounding the diagnosis and care of those with dementia. They provide an ethical framework for nursing those with a dementia and the care of their family that incorporates the humanising issues raised in this book and that will be further explored in Chapter 8.

Chapter summary

This chapter has explored the risk factors associated with dementia and recognised that addressing general healthy living activities will reduce the risk of developing dementia. Dementia was defined and then the major subtypes of dementia were described in order of prevalence: Alzheimer's, vascular, dementia with Lewy bodies, FTLD and CJD. The last two types of dementia examined were HIV and alcohol, both of which are considered reversible in some cases. It was acknowledged that the nurse's role in diagnosis and sharing was extremely important to facilitate a sense of well-being. The nurse's role was seen as primarily to support the person and their family, the best way to do this being through humanised person-centred care.

Activities: brief outline answers

Activity 6.1: Critical thinking (page 101)

To reduce your risk of developing diseases such as dementia, the general principles of healthy living apply.

- Diet – 'five a day', include fibre; avoid obesity.
- Exercise – regular physical exercise.
- Toxic substances – stay within government regulations for alcohol and salt intake; follow health safety guidelines on appliances; do not exceed recommended doses for medication.

- Stress management – make a little time for yourself each day and develop healthy coping strategies.
- Safe sex – minimise sexual partners and use condoms.
- Infection control – follow government guidelines 'catch it', 'bin it', 'kill it' and infection control policies.
- Regular health checks.

Activity 6.4: Critical thinking (page 111)

A diagnosis of dementia would have far-reaching effects for Neil. It will probably mean that he will have to stop paid employment, which will have an impact on his ability to pay his mortgage and provide for his children. He will lose the ability to drive his car. His children will probably be involved in caring for their father as he deteriorates. He will not be able to get certain types of insurance and may have problems taking family holidays overseas. As a nurse, you need to be aware of all these issues, and there may be many more, if you are to support him and his family so that they all retain a sense of well-being.

Activity 6.6: Critical thinking (page 119)

As in Neil's case, there are a number of areas that Mike and his family may need support with, and there are a number of agencies that you could guide Mike and his family towards to address their needs.

- The Alzheimer's Society – will offer support and guidance with information needs such as finances, diagnosis and practical support.
- Al-Anon – will continue to offer support and guidance.
- Social services – will help with carer's assessment and benefits advice.
- Dieticians – will ensure optimal nutritional diets.
- Care coordinator –will liaise and ensure interprofessional and interagency working.
- GP.

Further reading

Livingstone, G, Leavey, G, Manela, M, Livingston, D, Rait, G, Sampson, G, Barishi, S, Shahriyarmulki, K and Cooper, C (2010) Making decisions for people with dementia who lack capacity: qualitative study of family carers in UK. *BMJ*, 341: c4184.

This paper outlines some research undertaken on behalf of those with dementia and their carers on the various decisions that need to be made when a diagnosis of dementia has been made. Facts sheets for families can be found at: www.kirklees.gov.uk/community/care-support/partnerorgs/careinkirklees/workforce/DementiaFactsForCarers.pdf.

Nuffield Council on Bioethics (2009) Dementia: ethical issues. Cambridge: Cambridge Publishers.

This book offers more detailed information and guidance on the ethical dilemmas associated with a diagnosis of dementia.

Useful websites

http://alzheimers.org.uk/site/scripts/download_info.php?fileID=454

The *Out of the shadows* report in 2008 was developed from research undertaken to provide an understanding of the stigma and experiences of people and their families receiving a diagnosis of dementia.

http://dementia.dh.gov.uk/memory-assessment-service-specifications

The Department of Health's memory assessment service specifications web page sets out the expectations of services in their provision of memory assessments and sharing the diagnosis. It also gives links to good examples of services from a number of geographical areas.

www.aidsalliance.org

The International AIDS HIV Alliance is a global partnership of charities and organisations fighting HIV and building healthy communities. Its website offers a wide resource base for international information on AIDS and HIV.

www.al-anonuk.org.uk

The Al-anon and Alateen website provides links for support and information for family and friends who have been affected by alcohol abuse.

www.mndassociation.org

The Motor Neurone Disease Association offers information and advice on MND and explains research being undertaken in this area.

www.parkinsons.org.uk

Parkinson's UK offers information and support for those experiencing Parkinson's disease.

Chapter 7
Care

Introduction

Late in 2011 the BBC news carried a report that hospitals were ill equipped to deal with patients with dementia – one in four of all patients. This headline news was based on an audit report on the care for people with dementia that was conducted by the Royal College of Psychiatrists, the British Geriatrics Society, the Royal College of Nursing, the Royal College of Physicians, the Royal College of General Practitioners and the Alzheimer's Society. The audit was funded by the Healthcare Quality Improvement Partnership, and coordinated by the Royal College of Psychiatrists' Centre for Quality Improvement (CCQI). This report led to headlines such as *Hospital staff 'lack skills to cope with dementia patients'* (*Guardian*, 2011). The report highlighted that none of the NHS Trusts involved in the audit achieved all the essential standards of care.

This chapter focuses on the person-centred, humanising approach to care that we need in order to achieve the essential standards of care. It looks at current policies and reports that underpin service provision and the care environment. Last, it explores the available therapeutic nursing approaches, including medication and palliative care.

Supporting guidance

The Department of Health (DH) produced a report in 2009 called *Living well with dementia: a National Dementia Strategy* (DH, 2009); the dementia strategy implementation guide produced alongside this was revised in 2010 (DH, 2010a). These revisions were made to account for the White Paper *Equity and excellence: liberating the NHS* and *Liberating the NHS: transparency in outcomes*, which were introduced by the newly established Conservative–Liberal Democrat coalition (DH, 2010a).

The dementia strategy aimed to raise awareness of dementia in the general public, promote early diagnosis and intervention, and achieve a higher quality of care (DH, 2009, p9). To do this it provided 17 objectives that need to be implemented. The strategy offers a person-focused approach that incorporates the needs of carers along with objectives to develop services.

The National Institute for Health and Clinical Excellence (NICE) is a government body that sets the standards for high-quality health care and encourages healthy living (NICE, 2011a). It provided guidance for dementia care that was updated in 2011 to incorporate new evidence related to drug treatments; this will be considered later in the chapter. One of the main principles established by NICE is that dementia care should be given whenever possible at home. NICE also stated that it should be provided with respect for dignity, individual diversity and choice.

Both the DH and NICE developed their reports after consulting with people with dementia, their families and their carers. The reports can also be seen to have similar underpinning philosophical approaches. Along with these specific dementia care documents there has been the development of the Care Programme Approach (CPA) (DH, 2006) and the Single Assessment Process (SAP) (DH, 2001c). Both of these are used within mental health services: CPA provides a multi-professional care planning approach for people with complex needs to ensure comprehensive planning, implementation and evaluation, and SAP facilitates a reduction in the number of professionals the person needs to tell their story to (DH, 2005). CPA and SAP provide a person-centred approach with a recognition of the importance of family and carer.

Despite the availability of processes such as CPA and SAP, and guidance documents such as the dementia strategy and NICE guidelines, for many the experiences of dementia care is not a therapeutic one. The national audit referred to above, coordinated by the Royal College of Psychiatrists (RCPsych, 2011a), covered 99 per cent of the Trusts in England and Wales but found that none of the hospitals met all the essential standards for dementia care and that very few wards had a person-centred approach. Over two-thirds of the care staff in the hospitals said they felt they had inadequate training and skills to provide appropriate care for people with dementia.

The Nursing and Midwifery Council (NMC, 2011) states that, as nurses, we are accountable for our practice and we need to ensure we continually develop our knowledge and skills to provide care. This chapter should help guide you in your care of people with dementia and also enhance your understanding of the knowledge and skills you need to develop.

Medication

Although only a small number of nurses are prescribers, we all, at times, administer medication. We are accountable for our actions and therefore safe administration of medication, and to do this we need a good understanding of the therapeutic and non-therapeutic effects. An understanding of the mechanisms for their effect on the body is also helpful.

As was established in Chapter 6, there are a number of known and, to some extent, treatable causes of dementia, but for the most prevalent type of dementia – Alzheimer's dementia – there is no drug cure, although certain chemicals can slow down the progression of the disease for a period of time. Drug treatments of the different types of dementia could include:

- for Alzheimer's – cholinesterase inhibitors and NMDA (N-methyl-D-aspartate) receptor antagonists;
- for vascular – statins (to reduce cholesterol) and warfarin (anticoagulant – reduces the risk of clots forming) to address vascular problems, to ensure a good blood supply and to minimise the risk of strokes;
- for HIV – HAART to treat infection;
- for alcohol – alcohol consumption stopped and administration of vitamin B.

NICE (2011b) does not recommend the use of medication such as antipsychotics for behavioural and psychological symptoms associated with dementia (BPSD). The response to BPSD such as hallucinations or agitation should be other therapeutic techniques unless these have not been effective, the person is particularly distressed by them or they are at significant risk.

In Chapter 6 we considered diagnosis and also identified the biological processes that have been implicated in the development of dementia. Despite the research that has been undertaken, the evidence for a neuro-chemical explanation for dementia is inconclusive; however, there is enough evidence to support the therapeutic use of chemicals (medication) according to NICE (2011b). These medications are not a 'cure' as they only reduce deterioration and this reduction is usually time limited (Mutsatsa, 2011).

There are two main types of medication used to treat Alzheimer's disease – cholinesterase inhibitors and NMDA receptor antagonists – which work in different ways. Cholinesterase inhibitors include donepezil hydrochloride (Aricept), rivastigmine (Exelon) and galantamine (Reminyl). These are indicated for mild to moderate Alzheimer's, whereas the NMDA receptor antagonist memantine (Ebixa) is recommended for moderate to severe Alzheimer's (NICE, 2011b).

Donepezil hydrochloride was the first drug to be licensed in the UK specifically for Alzheimer's disease, and memantine is the newest of the Alzheimer's drugs. In Alzheimer's disease, evidence shows that there is a loss of nerve cells that use a chemical called acetylcholine as a chemical messenger (a neurotransmitter). The degree of loss of these nerve cells is related to the severity of symptoms that people experience.

Donepezil hydrochloride, rivastigmine and galantamine prevent the enzyme acetylcholinesterase from breaking down acetylcholine in the brain. Increased concentrations of acetylcholine lead to increased communication between the nerve cells that use acetylcholine. This may temporarily improve or stabilise the symptoms of Alzheimer's disease, and may help slow decline. All three cholinesterase inhibitors work in a similar way, but one might suit an individual better than another, particularly in terms of side effects experienced (Alzheimer's Society, 2011b).

Memantine is an NMDA receptor antagonist that stops the increased glutamate in synapses from binding to the NMDA receptors in the brain. The damage to nerve cells (neurones) caused by beta amyloidal proteins through plaques and tangles increases the amount of glutamate in the synapse (see Chapter 6). This excessive glutamate interferes with the chemical message being transmitted across the synapse, leading to symptoms of Alzheimer's. Memantine blocks the effect of excessive glutamate and allows the messages to continue from one neurone to another. It has been suggested that this drug can also help people with dementia with Lewy bodies, but there is still more research needed with these drugs (NICE, 2011b).

Dementias caused by vascular disease, HIV and alcohol should have their causes treated by the appropriate drug therapies or other interventions, but any residual symptoms will need other approaches. While NICE recognises the usefulness of drugs to treat the symptoms of Alzheimer's disease, it also recommends the use of other therapies such as aromatherapy, massage, music, multi-sensory stimulation and animal therapy (NICE, 2011b). Other available therapies will be considered later in this chapter.

Assistive technologies

Assistive technologies are devices or systems that can help a person with dementia remain as independent as possible despite reduced ability. Assistive technologies (ATs) can be simple devices such as notepads, diaries and calendars, but can also involve telecare items such as detectors of gas, smoke or falls. The Alzheimer's Society states that ATs can be accessed that support:

- speaking;
- hearing;
- eyesight;
- moving about;
- getting out and about;
- memory;
- cognition;
- daily living activities;
- socialising.

For each of these areas there are a number of devices available. Those highlighted by the Alzheimer's Society include memory devices, telecare and devices to enable safer walking. There are, of course, a wide range of devices to support the health care problems associated with dementia as well. For example, devices are available to reduce the problems of urinary or faecal incontinence, which can be very embarrassing for the person. As nurses, we need to be aware of the availability of these devices. Occupational therapists and physiotherapists have access to appropriate devices and will be able to guide the person with dementia to what would be most helpful for them. The Alzheimer's Society will also offer guidance (see Useful websites at the end of the chapter).

There are many small assistive technologies that we, as nurses, can use to give our patients with dementia greater independence. Many have problems with their depth perception and distinguishing between patterns, which can create problems moving around and undertaking everyday tasks. We can organise the environment to reduce confusion and enhance a sense of well-being.

- Removal of rugs and mats are generally considered a hazard for tripping, but they can also be perceived to be steps and the person might try to step up or down on to them.
- Shiny surfaces can appear to be surfaces covered with water, and the person may be unhappy to walk across them; they can appear to be less shiny with small changes to the lighting.
- The use of plain tablecloths can allow the person to more clearly see their plate and cutlery as patterned ones make them more difficult to distinguish.
- Colour coding of doors or the hanging of names or pictures on them can help the person to identify which door they need to use.

These are just a few small examples of how, as nurses using our observational and problem solving skills, we can use assistive technology to support people living with dementia.

Reality orientation

Reality orientation (RO) has been an approach used within mental health and older persons' services for a number of years and was initially seen as a useful tool in caring for people with dementia. While it is still seen as useful, it is recognised as limited, as the case study shows.

Case study: Melissa

Melissa is 80 years old. Her parents died a long time ago, and her husband died eight years ago. Melissa has Alzheimer's dementia and is in residential care. At times she becomes confused and disorientated, usually when her carer has asked her to do something, for example, come to the table for her meal. When Melissa is confused she cries and asks for her mother. Using a reality orientation approach, the carer explains to Melissa that her mother, father and husband are dead.

Activity 7.1	*Critical thinking*

Read the case of Melissa. Why do you think using reality orientation in this situation might not be appropriate?

An outline answer is given at the end of the chapter.

RO as provided to Melissa in the case study may be considered to be unethical, since it may cause her further distress every time she hears it, although to lie to her could also be considered unethical. RO can, though, be a very useful tool. It can be used in two ways: formal and informal. A formal method of using RO could be in a group setting where a few people with dementia get together and consider the day, date, season or things that are happening on the television or in the newspapers.

An informal approach is usually used as part of everyday care; for example, each time a carer interacts with the person with dementia they inform them of pertinent information. This can be quite demoralising for the carer, though, if they have explained to the person with dementia that it is 'Tuesday the 4th of February' ten times during the morning.

Orientation to reality is seen as essential if a person is to make decisions about their lives, so while it can cause problems, nurses need to be able to use this approach. RO and AT, as with other therapeutic approaches, require a clear philosophy of care to be established, as we have already recognised. The dementia care strategy and NICE guidelines lead us to work in a person-centred way, supporting the person's family and carers. Tom Kitwood developed this dialectical approach, called person-centred care, for dementia care in the 1980s. He argued that the person with dementia is not just a victim to their bodies; they are interacting with others and their environment and he found these to be exacerbating the problems experienced. He found that the care environment was characterised by malignant social psychology; to provide appropriate care, nurses needed to exhibit positive person work.

Positive person work

Positive person work was introduced in Chapter 3, where we identified how caring for a person with dementia could become malignant social psychology but that positive person work would make care more person-centred and therapeutic. Positive person work involves recognition, negotiation, collaboration, play, **timalation**, **celebration**, relaxation, validation, holding and facilitation. These terms were introduced in Chapter 3, but we will look at them now in more detail.

Recognition – for example, welcoming the person by name – can demonstrate respect and acknowledgement that the person is an individual who deserves to be treated as such. Welcoming can be an important activity for a person who is struggling with their memory and may be confused. To welcome the person by name orientates them to who they are; introducing yourself, and mentioning the reason for the meeting, can help facilitate a sense of control rather than confusion.

Negotiation and collaboration can also foster a sense of control and self-respect. If the person's choices, opinions and feelings are respected by others, it aids their sense of themselves as deserving of respect. Malignant social psychology, on the other hand, encourages dependence and self-deprecation, which can lead to low self-esteem, anxiety and depression.

Play and timalation provide time and opportunity for pleasure. A person with dementia needs to be cared for in a manner that encourages them to feel a sense of worth through time for play and timalation, but enjoying an activity can also boost the person's sense of well-being.

Celebration – for example, taking the opportunity to express pleasure together in seeing a small child play – is recognised by nurses as relevant and an important interaction; it can also validate the person. Validation of how the person is feeling is so significant that it has become a therapeutic approach and is discussed later in this chapter.

Relaxation is a necessary part of care; people need to be offered time and an environment where they do not feel pressured. Pressure and stress can affect health in a negative way. For a lot of people relaxation occurs when they are alone, but in positive person work this needs to be undertaken with another person, such as a nurse. The nurse needs to sit quietly with the person, respecting their stillness, but at the same time providing a reassuring presence.

For the professional nurse, touch and holding has become a difficult part of care, as professional distance and boundaries are part of their syllabus. If nurses struggle with therapeutic touch such as holding, most do not struggle ethically with touch to perform physical interventions; nurses need to discuss these boundaries with their mentor or clinical supervisor. When Kitwood (1997) writes about holding, he does not just mean touch; he also means giving the person the space to express their feelings.

The last of Kitwood's positive person work is facilitation, which is probably the element that nurses find themselves most drawn to do automatically. Facilitation is about providing the personal resources to allow the person to undertake something they wish to do. This could be as simple as putting their coat on or as complex as providing picture mats or electronic software so that they can communicate with others.

All of Kitwood's positive person work is about ensuring the highest quality of life through the person having personal control and the facilitation of self-esteem and a sense of well-being.

As was first explained in Chapter 2, there are other, newer approaches that can be used in dementia care nursing, so while positive person work is accepted as facilitating high-quality care, humanising this care can further improve a sense a well-being in the person, and it is this approach that we examine now.

Humanising care

Kitwood's person-centred approach to dementia care has its roots in humanistic psychology. This is also true for Todres et al. (2009) along with the recognition of a biomedical element, but whereas Kitwood incorporated a sociological influence, Todres et al. take a view of the person from existential phenomenological perspective or a philosophical approach. Kitwood may be seen to be bio-psycho-social in approach, whereas Todres et al. may be seen as applying a philosophical understanding to care.

Although humanistic psychology was briefly described in Chapter 4, it is worth considering a couple of the humanistic psychologists here in a little more detail, along with the philosophical position of the phenomenologists.

Abraham Maslow (1908–1970), a humanist psychologist, provided us with 'a hierarchy of needs' in which the person addresses the lowest level of need before being able to progress to higher needs. Those needs at the bottom of the hierarchy are referred to as deficiency needs and the higher ones as growth needs. If deficiency needs are unresolved, the person becomes unwell, but if growth needs are not met, the person will not reach self-actualisation (their potential).

Deficiency needs are:

- physiological;
- safety;
- love and belonging;
- esteem.

Growth needs are:

- cognitive;
- aesthetic;
- self-actualisation.

Carl Ransom Rogers (1902–1987) developed a humanistic theory of the person recognising their uniqueness and need for self-actualisation, but also the need for positive regard from others. His client-centred therapy provided a space where people could work things out for themselves in a supportive environment; they had the opportunity to grow into themselves. The therapy was non-directive, but the therapist offered non-judgemental positive regard for the person. Most professional counselling is based on these principles.

For both Rogers and Maslow the person is unique and has the potential to reach self-actualisation, but to achieve this they need to develop and grow within a social context. The person is seen as able to make their own choices and fulfil their own destiny. These theories form part of the work of Kitwood and Todres et al.

The experiences of the person described by the humanists have similarities with the philosophical approach of Edmund Husserl's notion of lifeworld. Husserl and those who followed him (Heidegger, Merleau-Ponty) – with their concepts of embodiment, **temporality**, **spatiality**, human freedom, **ownness**, body subject, body object – all influenced the development of the humanising care approach of Todres et al. (2009).

The philosophically informed framework Todres et al. developed to humanise care incorporates the concepts of:

- uniqueness;
- personal journey;
- agency;
- insiderness;
- togetherness;
- embodiment;
- sense making;
- sense of place.

See Chapter 2 for more explanation. We can use an appreciation of these concepts alongside a knowledge of the positive person work developed from Kitwood's person-centred care to ensure the broadest approach to care for people with dementia. The person-centred care approach of Kitwood and the humanising of care are the underpinning philosophy of care advocated in this book.

Activities of daily living

The definition given in the dementia strategy (DH, 2009) clearly states that to have dementia causes the person to have problems with daily activities. The type of activity first affected will depend on where the brain cell death occurs, but as dementia is a progressive disorder, all activities will eventually be affected. Roper et al. (1980) outlined what are considered to be the activities of daily living in their model of nursing care. The assessment, planning, implementation and evaluation of the care to support a person's ability to achieve their daily activities, according to Roper et al. (1980), must take into consideration context (psychological, social, environmental, political, lifespan stage and influencing factors) and the level of independence of the person. The activities of daily living (Roper et al., 1980) are:

- maintaining a safe environment;
- communication;
- breathing;
- eating and drinking;

- eliminating;
- personal cleansing and dressing;
- controlling body temperature;
- mobilising;
- working and playing;
- expressing sexuality;
- sleeping;
- dying.

To offer nursing care for any of these activities we must consider individual differences and preferences respecting personhood. If we undertake our nursing care using a person-centred and humanising approach, we can maintain the person's sense of themselves and their self-esteem, which will facilitate a sense of well-being.

Case study: Myra McCarthy

Myra was diagnosed with Alzheimer's dementia eight years ago. Over the eight years the progression of her dementia has been gradual and steady. Gaining a diagnosis was a fraught time for her and her husband, but when they received the diagnosis they took lots of advice and received support from the Alzheimer's Society, her GP and the newly established memory clinic. Myra organised all her legal and financial affairs while she still had mental capacity to do so, and her husband now has lasting power of attorney. A year ago Myra's personal care needs became too much for her husband and she moved to a nursing home for people with dementia. Over the first few weeks Myra's condition deteriorated significantly, but with compassionate nursing care Myra has shown little distress and her husband can see signs of comfort and contentment in her eyes.

When assessing and planning Myra's care, Roper et al.'s activities of daily living were taken into consideration along with the needs established by Kitwood and Maslow. Achievement of Myra's needs was supported by nurses taking into account positive person work and Todres et al.'s humanising agenda.

Maintaining a safe environment – *Myra is unable to manage her external environment and has limited independence with her internal environment. Nursing staff therefore have to be vigilant and to notice any cues that Myra is uncomfortable or is at risk of harm. As her mobility is limited, they also need to monitor and provide pressure area care.*

Communication – *Myra is able to indicate how she is feeling through ill-defined limb and eye movements; she will also make noises that can be interpreted as discomfort or pleasure. Nurses need to closely observe for any attempts by Myra to communicate; if they are unsure of the meaning of a gesture or noise made by her, they are to discuss it with her husband. Nurses are expected to communicate both verbally and non-verbally with Myra during all interactions with her.*

Breathing – *Myra has a long history of asthma, so at times she has problems with her breathing; the nurses administer salbutamol through a nebuliser. In her advance directive on treatment Myra wanted this therapy to continue to alleviate the distress of struggling to breathe, but she did not want any associated illnesses treated except with pain relief.*

continued . . .

Eating and drinking – *Myra is able to indicate if she does not want the food offered to her, and her husband has given the nurses a list of her preferred food and drinks. Usually Myra's husband feeds her as this allows him to feel involved and Myra eats more when he is there. Nurses need to support Myra's husband with her care. If nurses need to feed Myra, humming or singing at the same time has facilitated her eating.*

Eliminating – *Myra is able to give non-verbal cues about her need to empty her bowels; she fidgets in her chair. However, she does not appear to be aware of the need to pass urine; she wears incontinence pads.*

Personal cleansing and dressing – *Myra does appear to be aware of the clothes that are offered to her to wear, and her husband is sure she indicates which she prefers each day. Usually her husband will organise the clothes she is to wear the next day with her, but if he has not done this, nurses need to involve Myra in this decision. Myra is unable to wash or dress herself, but she is more relaxed when being washed and dressed when music is played and when each small step of the interventions is explained and consent is requested.*

Controlling body temperature – *Myra is unable to dress herself so she is unable to manage her temperature by putting on or taking off clothes. Nurses need to be mindful of this and check verbally as well as observing for non-verbal cues of discomfort.*

Mobilising – *Myra has some movement in her limbs, but this appears uncoordinated at times. She is unable to walk, but she can stand with support. A hoist needs to be used to move Myra on to the toilet and her bed. This can distress Myra, but humming or singing helps her relax when this needs to be done.*

Working and playing – *Myra enjoyed singing madrigals, gardening and needlework, and appears to be more relaxed when she is in the garden or singing. She is able to join in with the songs her husband sings to her, although the words are indistinguishable to others.*

Expressing sexuality – *Both Myra and her husband get pleasure in being together, whether they are sitting quietly holding hands or engaged in an activity.*

Sleeping – *Myra has been spending increasing amounts of time sleeping. She sleeps most of the night despite disturbances to check if she has been incontinent, and she has a morning and afternoon nap.*

Dying – *When they were given the diagnosis Myra and her husband discussed how her dying and death should be managed. Both of them felt it was better to have quality of life, and Myra has written an advance directive stating that if her heart or breathing was to fail, she should be allowed to die. She was also fearful of being in pain and no one noticing; she would prefer to be over-medicated than to be in pain.*

Activity 7.2   *Critical thinking*

Read the case study of Myra McCarthy and identify ways in which personhood and humanised care have been enacted.

An outline answer is provided at the end of the chapter.

The case study of Myra provides a very brief example of how an ongoing holistic assessment and care planning can be developed in a humanised manner using positive person work.

There are a number of therapies available to support and enhance the person's ability to undertake their activities of daily living and for them to gain a sense of well-being. Using the humanising and person-centred approach to care giving, we need to ensure the therapeutic approach addresses the individual needs of the person and those they are in relationship with. To undertake any of these, though, we need to develop good communication skills; we need to communicate in creative ways.

Creative communication

Communication can involve verbal and non-verbal techniques. Most nurses use verbal techniques in a conscious manner, but nurses who are good at communication observe and use non-verbal techniques as well; this was initially described in Chapter 5.

Killick and Allen (2001) state that there are a number of ways in which to enhance communication with people who have dementia. They include: 'stopping talking', body language including mirroring, pacing, going with the flow, completing utterances (just a few words), communicating during other activities, gaining trust and self-disclosure. These skills relate closely to the basic communication skills discussed in Chapter 5, such as Rogers' effective communication and Egan's SOLER.

Some very practical advice by Adams (2008, pp146, 147) on how to develop good communication in dementia care nursing is set out in the theory summary box.

Theory summary: Adams's communication

Attracting attention
- Say the person's name, gain eye contact and speak directly to them.

Maintaining attention
- Use appropriate gestures such as gently touching the person's arm.

Verbal techniques
- Use short simple sentences: speak slowly and clearly with easy-to-understand sentences.
- Repeat sentences or change words with ones with the same meaning if the person does not seem to understand.
- Be specific.
- Do not say *Don't you remember?*
- Offer simple choices – closed questions.
- Give instructions one step at a time.

Non-verbal techniques
- Use labels that can be words or pictures.
- Use signals – touching an arm, pointing to things, body language (smiling, frowning etc.).
- Listen – use reflection and paraphrasing.
- Give time for the person to answer.
- Reduce distractions.

As nurses, we need to listen using all of our senses so that we have all the available information about how the person is feeling and what they may want or need. Likewise, we need to use all of our communication skills to engage with people with dementia. Activity 7.3 will help you consider the breadth of your communication skills.

Activity 7.3   Reflection

Identify as many different ways as possible that you communicate with other people.

An outline answer is provided at the end of the chapter.

As you found in Activity 7.3, there are a huge number of ways in which you communicate with others; as long as there is a connection between you and another person there will be communication. Some people believe that even when there is a great distance and no physical connection (telephones, satellite communication etc.) between themselves and a loved one, they still know how they are feeling.

Creative communication can be used as a means to provide care, but it can also be a therapeutic activity in the same way as other activities, such as reminiscence therapy. You can use a variety of media such as pictures and stories – in particular, using life stories has become a major element of dementia care nursing. Collecting life story information, especially when it is supported by pictures and other objects, can facilitate positive person work and humanised care. A nurse who has a record of the person's life story can engage with the person on a much more intimate level; it helps the person to recognise themselves as a unique person with individual experiences and relationships. The use of life story boxes and books has many similarities to reminiscence work, and this is the next therapeutic approach to be considered here.

Reminiscence therapy

Reminiscence is seen as a valuable activity to maintain mental health, especially for older people. It allows the person to recognise their achievements and revisit significant events. Reminiscence can facilitate an understanding of where the person 'fits in'; it helps them make sense of their experiences and can promote positive spirituality (see Chapter 3 for further discussion of spirituality).

It would appear paradoxical that a memory-based therapy is used to help those with memory problems – using 'weakness as strength' – but reminiscence therapy has developed significantly over the last 15 years. It was used in mental health services before this time, but today it is recognised that it can be used in a wide variety of situations.

Reminiscence therapy is usually conducted in group situations where the other members of the group can prompt and facilitate further exploration of the individual experience. Sharing experiences can fulfil a number of the humanistic needs identified by Maslow and by Kitwood (1993) along with the virtues of Erikson and the senses of Nolan et al. (2004). Alongside these attributes, reminiscence can be seen to be a humanising approach to care (Todres et al., 2009).

Reminiscence can be prompted in many ways. Nurses working with this approach have used a wide variety of tools, including music, objects to handle or smell and pictures; some have even taken the person into a situation such as a public house or a theatre. Some residential settings have set up sensory rooms, where patients can feel, hear, smell, see certain experiences such as the seaside, with the room set up like a beach, with sand on the floor and sea sounds in the background.

Case study: Jane

Jane is a student nurse working alongside an occupational therapist in a day unit for people with moderate dementia. The occupational therapist usually facilitates a reminiscence group once a week for a group of men. As part of her placement with the day unit Jane has worked alongside a number of other professionals as well as her nurse mentor. Jane has enjoyed the reminiscence group, and this week she has been given the opportunity to lead the group. Jane has put a lot of effort into preparation. As the men are all over 70 years old and have lived in the UK all their lives, they all experienced the Second World War and rationing of food. Jane has collected together items such as pictures of the food available at that time, ration books and a gas mask.

Jane starts the session by asking the men if they recognise the items. The men do indeed remember the items and give examples of when and where they came into contact with them. This provokes other memories of the war, their education and teachers, and their mothers cooking. Jane is left with the impression that their mothers were poor cooks, but at the debriefing with the occupational therapist afterwards she learns that these women had to cope with few of the ingredients and tools available today. The men appear to enjoy the session, and for a couple their frequently mask-like faces brighten with recognition and reliving of pleasurable moments.

Reminiscence allows both the nurse and the person to recognise personhood and the establishment of compassion and respect. This can facilitate the validation of the person promoted by both Kitwood and Todres et al.

Validation therapy

Validation therapy is about recognising how the person is feeling, and accepting and responding to this even if we as nurses do not think it is the most appropriate way to feel.

Techniques that can be used in validation therapy (Adams, 2008, p166) include:

- centring;
- building trust through use of factual words: what, when, where, why, how;
- rephrasing;
- using polarity;
- imaging the opposite;
- reminiscing;
- maintaining genuine close eye contact;
- using ambiguity;
- using clear, low, loving tone of voice;
- mirroring – observing and matching the person's behaviour and emotions;
- linking behaviour with unmet needs;
- identifying and using the person's preferred sense: hearing, touch, sight, etc.;
- using music.

Read the case study about Paul to gain a better understanding of how these terms can be put into practice.

Case study: Paul

*Paul is a student nurse who has been visiting Mr Peter Wright for a couple of weeks with the community nurse. Mr Wright has complex needs that include dementia; he is no longer in employment but he was headmaster of a public school for boys and he lives at home with his wife. Paul has observed the community nurse interacting with Mr Wright, and on this occasion Paul has been asked to assess any changes in Mr Wright's well-being. Paul and the nurse are invited into the sitting room where Mr Wright stands to meet them. Paul takes a deep breath (**centring** himself), shakes the offered hand and says 'Hello' to Mr Wright, using his name, introduces himself and explains why he is there.*

*Mr Wright invites Paul to sit down; Paul does so and accepts a cup of coffee from Mrs Wright. Paul sits near to Mr Wright and gains eye contact with him. They share the paperwork that needs to be completed, and Paul asks him in a clear, caring, low tone how the past week has been for him. Mr Wright complains that his sight is not good and is causing him a problem so Paul focuses on giving and receiving information verbally (**preferred sense**).*

*Mr Wright's voice becomes thick and he struggles with words; his wife says it has been a difficult week. As Mr Wright leans forward and hugs his abdomen Paul leans forward also (**mirroring**) and asks Do you have pain in your abdomen? (**linking behaviour**). Mr Wright indicates that he does. Paul appears concerned (mirroring) and asks him how long he has been in pain (factual words). Mr Wright says he cannot remember but it is a long time. Paul asks if he has any pain anywhere else and Mr Wright is able to indicate a couple of other areas of his body.*

*Paul continues to lean forward, mirroring Mr Wright's posture, and asks if he has had pain like this before (**reminiscing**). As Mr Wright explains the pain he has had before and the context of it, Paul rephrases (**rephrasing**) what has been said to ensure he has understood and to validate Mr Wright's explanation. Paul slowly builds up a picture of Mr Wright's condition using mirroring, verbal and non-verbal communication skills, reminiscing and observing his behaviour.*

The case study of Paul demonstrates how techniques you probably use in your everyday interaction can facilitate validation and can therefore be easily used in your nursing care. There are, though, other therapeutic activities that need extra organisation, such as art therapy.

Art therapy

The importance of art such as painting and drawing as an educational tool, spiritual activity and enjoyable pastime has been recognised since Neolithic times. Art has been used by children and adults alike, but it has also been seen as a way of accessing a person's thoughts and feelings when they are unable to put them into words.

A man with vascular dementia said to Baines (2008, p110): *creativity is the essence of life. If you think about it, all life is creative.*

The use of art therapy for those with dementia is a more recent intervention. It has been recognised that although a person with dementia may have lost verbal speech, they may retain the ability to recognise and draw items that are important to them. Art therapy can increase self-esteem by providing a means of communication and pleasure in the activity, but also by providing the opportunity to interact more closely with their carers. Art therapists aim to empower people who feel they have lost their creativeness to regain their abilities and raise self-worth. Baines (2008) draws on theories of neural plasticity and how, despite brain cell death, there is still the opportunity for other areas of the brain to adapt and continue creativity.

Art therapy is not about developing an accurate drawing of an object, but is about the freedom to paint or draw without concern that what is created is right or wrong, good or bad; this can be determined only by the person who has created it. Some therapists use the artwork to create the space to talk and interact with others, but they all acknowledge the power of creation itself.

Music therapy

Music therapy can reach the person with dementia at a deeper level than spoken words alone. Music can offer the person a sense of place and help them engage with thoughts, feelings and memories not accessible by other routes. It can stimulate the brain and ignite the spirit. Evidence suggests that people with dementia retain their music ability when other forms of communication and social skills are lost (Robertson-Gillam, 2011). There are generally considered to be two forms of music therapy: one uses music to support other therapies; the other uses music by itself.

As was seen in the case study of Myra McCarthy, music and singing can reduce distress and enhance the care-giving experience. Caregivers singing as part of personal care has been found to reduce aggressive responses (Adams, 2008) and enhance the person's ability to engage in independent care. Singing is the most potent communication skill available to people with dementia (Robertson-Gillam, 2011). It has been found to relieve stress, facilitate relaxation, reduce physiological tension and enhance communication (Adams, 2008).

Dance therapy

Dance therapy has the therapeutic advantages of music therapy, but also engages with the music in a more active way. It can be seen as a method of reminiscence, as memories are not just semantic in nature; they can also be **procedural** – the memory of how to do something. Reminiscence therapy can facilitate the remembering of who the person is and their previous experiences, thus reinforcing self-identity and self-concept. Dance therapy can, though, offer something more: it offers the reliving – the embodiment – of the person they were and are, which can more fully facilitate self-esteem and a holistic sense of well-being. The case study of Derrick Joyce will help with your understanding of this.

Case study: Derrick Joyce

Derrick has severe dementia and cannot move around independently; he is confined to a wheelchair and he is mute. Derrick and his wife attended church services every week and enjoyed the social activities associated with it. Derrick had a robust singing voice and enjoyed all types of music with the exception of what he considered the 'loud banging' music that young people liked.

Derrick developed dementia after retirement. Initially, he became forgetful but his wife compensated for this. After some time he gradually became unable to wash and dress himself to his usual standard. There were also occasions when Derrick was found to be missing, and searches had to be made for him. He gradually lost the ability to verbally communicate, and his face became immobile.

Despite the difficulties, Derrick's family ensured he retained most of the activities he had undertaken before his deterioration. He attended church every week and all the church social events. Derrick's family organised for him to attend the Harvest Festival barn dance. Initially, Derrick did not seem to notice what was happening around him as he sat passively in his wheelchair but Derrick's carers were encouraged to push the wheelchair in time with the music among the dancers. As Derrick moved in time with the music there appeared to be a flicker of response in his eyes, and as the women twirled round him from one partner to the next Derrick held their hand with his left hand and then passed it to his right. He was dancing!

In the case study of Derrick Joyce, you can see that, despite his advanced dementia, through dance Derrick is able to engage with others and the person he is in a more embodied way.

Dance therapy can also be undertaken as a therapeutic group activity, allowing the people involved to relive and make new enjoyable moments. It can enhance the ability to communicate with others and for some even reawaken speech: *the body is used as a substitute or as a support to speech* (Adams, 2008, p172).

There are a vast number of therapies available, and the number is further increased by the different ways in which people use or interact with them. Other examples are drama, aromatherapy, massage, *snoezelen*, cognitive behavioural therapy, psychodynamic therapy and animal therapy.

For some, the more concrete approaches, such as cognitive behavioural therapy and reality orientation, are the most suitable, but for others the more aesthetic and spiritual approaches are beneficial. It is important that we gather life stories and understand the life world experiences of the person in order to help us identify what would be most appropriate.

For all people the inevitable conclusion to life is death, but for the person with dementia their progression to death is generally limited and more predictable. It has been suggested that palliative care should begin at diagnosis.

Palliative care

The term 'palliative' comes from the Latin word *palliare*, which means 'to cloak'; this relates closely to the definition the World Health Organization provides for palliative care, which is care that:

> *improves the quality of life of patients and their families facing the problem associated with life-threatening illness, through the prevention and relief of suffering by means of early identification and impeccable assessment and treatment of pain and other problems, physical, psychosocial and spiritual.*
> (WHO, 2012)

The National Council for Palliative Care (NCPC) offers the following definition of palliative care:

> *it embraces many elements of supportive care. It has been defined by NICE as follows:*

> *Palliative care is the active holistic care of patients with advanced progressive illness. Management of pain and other symptoms and provision of psychological, social and spiritual support is paramount. The goal of palliative care is achievement of the best quality of life for patients and their families. Many aspects of palliative care are also applicable earlier in the course of the illness in conjunction with other treatments.*
> (NCPC, 2012)

As can be seen from these definitions, a person with dementia should be able to access palliative care as soon as they receive a diagnosis, but they may not wish to see their condition as palliative until their abilities to undertake daily living activities decline.

Initiatives have developed to ensure that palliative care is available for people with dementia from diagnosis until death. NICE and SCIE (2006) have identified 12 key principles for palliative care for people with dementia that address the aims for palliative care. People with dementia can expect to have appropriate pain relief, given in their own home, and support with making decisions before they lack the competence to do so. Standards have been developed to address their care needs, which include the Gold Standards Framework (GSF), the Liverpool Care Pathway (LCP) and Preferred Priorities of Care (PPC) (NHS, 2012). These three sets of standards can be summarised as follows.

- GSF – focuses on continuity, communication and coordination.
- LCP – focuses on the end of life, the last 48–72 hours, and aims to achieve a pain-free death while addressing the holistic needs of person and their family.
- PPC – focuses on finding out the preferences of the person and their family.

The strategy, policies and standards indicated here are all consistent with providing a person-centred, humanising approach to dementia nursing care. The research so far, though, does not indicate that all people with dementia are receiving this type of care (Downs and Bowers, 2008; RCPsych, 2011a), so it is our aim, supported by government policy and research evidence, to promote a person-centred, humanised approach to care accessing the palliative care programme.

> ## Chapter summary
>
> This chapter has taken you on a journey to discover how you can provide optimal care for people with dementia. It has progressed from considering the policies and reports that are available to guide dementia care (DH, 2009; NICE, 2011b) through a consideration of medical responses, including medication and assistive technologies, to more aesthetic approaches of art, music and dance therapy, to its conclusion with palliative care. Whichever therapeutic approach – or mixture of approaches – is taken, it needs to be provided in a person-centred, humanised manner, offering respect and compassion for the person.

Activities: brief outline answers

Activity 7.1: Critical thinking (page 128)

Each time the nurse informs Melissa that the people she loves are dead she goes through the trauma of receiving the information as a first time. This could be considered ethically unacceptable as it is not behaving in a non-maleficent manner. The nurse causes Melissa pain by doing this. While it would also be unethical to lie, there are other techniques that can be used in this situation – for example, identifying what has caused her distress and creating comfort for her.

Activity 7.2: Critical thinking (page 133)

The elements of positive person work are incorporated in the assessment and care given to Myra; she is *recognised* as a person through her individuality, **validating** her self-concept, and her care as far as is possible is **negotiated** with her. The nurse works with Myra and her husband, *collaboratively facilitating* time for *play, celebration and relaxation*. The nurses also facilitate the opportunity for Myra and her husband to *hold* each other and gain *timalation* through touch.

The nurses are providing care in a humanised way by acknowledging and attempting to comply with Myra and her husband's advance directives. This respects the *uniqueness* of the individual, their *personal journey* and *agency*. *Insiderness* is recognised through these, too, but also through their attempts to interpret the non-verbal cues Myra gives and her clothes and food choices. The nurses offer *togetherness* themselves but also in the support of Myra's husband. *Embodiment* is demonstrated in the respectful way in which Myra's physical body is cared for alongside her relationships, as they are all part of Myra's experience of herself in the world. The nurses and Myra's husband help Myra *make sense* of her experiences and gain a *sense of place* by being with her and by their interactions such as singing, providing her comfort.

Activity 7.3: Reflection (page 135)

There are many ways in which you communicate with others. Here is a short list that may guide your recognition of some of the channels you use.

- Verbal face to face.
- Sign language.
- PowerPoint presentations.
- Posters.
- Facebook.
- MSN messenger.
- Acting things out, such as charades, role modelling.
- Writing.
- Drawing/painting.
- Sculpting.
- Touch – hugging, kissing, massage, stroking.
- Singing.
- Dancing.
- Pointing/showing.
- Pulling faces, frowning, smiling, pouting, blowing kisses.
- Hand gestures – V for victory sign, saluting.

Further reading

James, O (2008) *Contented dementia*. London: Vermillion.

This book offers strategies on caring for someone with dementia. It could also be recommended to relatives of those with dementia to help them develop their own care strategies.

Lee, H and Adams, T (2011) *Creative approaches in dementia care*. Basingstoke: Palgrave.

This book offers an evidence-based exploration of a number of non-medical therapeutic approaches to caring for people with dementia. The therapeutic approaches include some of those mentioned in this chapter in more detail and others that there has not been room to consider here.

Useful websites

http://publications.nice.org.uk/dementia-cg42/guidance

These are the NICE guidelines for dementia care.

www.atdementia.org.uk/editorial.asp?page_id=45

The AT Dementia website provides information and advice on assistive technologies for people with dementia. There are also a number of case studies on this site to allow you a better understanding of how they can facilitate independence. It also provides a self-assessment guide.

www.endoflifecareforadults.nhs.uk/strategy

The NHS End of Life Care website has been developed for health care professionals such as nurses and provides the policies and strategies for end-of-life care to which people with dementia are entitled. It offers case studies to improve your understanding of the principles.

Chapter 8
The legal and ethical context

continued . . . ●●

By entry to register:

v. Works within legal frameworks when seeking consent.

vii. Demonstrates respect for the autonomy and rights of people to withhold consent in relation to treatment within legal frameworks and in relation to people's safety.

Cluster: Organisational aspects of care

11. People can trust the newly registered graduate nurse to safeguard children and adults from vulnerable situations and support and protect them from harm.

Cluster: Medicines management

34. People can trust the newly registered graduate nurse to work within legal and ethical frameworks that underpin safe and effective medicines management.

Chapter aims

On completion of this chapter you should have developed an understanding of:

- ethical decision-making;
- the legalisation available to protect vulnerable people such as those with dementia.

Introduction

In January 2012 a report chaired by Lord Falconer suggested there should be a change in the legalisation on assisted dying, which is currently illegal. This caused a great deal of media coverage of the issue, with people taking opposing positions. Some people felt that assisted dying is immoral and should remain illegal, but others felt that if the person wishes to die and has the capacity to say so, they should be helped to end their life with dignity, just as they would with any other activity. As nurses, we need to engage in these ethical and legal debates as we will not only be involved in advocating for the autonomy of the person but also be called upon to provide assistance if the law is changed.

This chapter looks at the most significant legislation that will concern you in dementia care nursing. First, it will explore the guidance available to you when you have to make moral decisions as a nurse.

The ethical context

In nursing, we face many situations where a decision needs to be made that can be considered a moral or ethical issue. Consider some of the examples in Activity 8.1.

Activity 8.1   *Reflection*

How would you respond to these requests from patients?

- *I know I have diabetes but could you get me some chocolate from the shop? It would really cheer me up.*
- *Don't tell anyone, but you have been really kind to me so I bought you this present.*
- *My daughter is coming to see me today and I can't face seeing her. Could you tell her I have gone for tests or something?*

How would these situations make you feel?

As this is a personal reflection, there is no outline answer at the end of the chapter.

The primary source of guidance we have as nurses is our code of conduct (NMC, 2011). This clearly outlines the behaviour expected of us. Our professional body has other supplementary guides for different areas of our work, such as record keeping, gifts and whistle blowing. There are also our contracts of employment, and policies and procedures set by our employers. The guidance and advice given by these organisations are based on the available evidence but are influenced by the pervading culture, just like our personal moral decision-making.

Activity 8.2   *Reflection*

This activity is not about your actual views, but about what brings you to have those views. It might be the way you were brought up (that is, your family's values), your religious beliefs or the result of rational decision-making. Take a few minutes to think about what has affected your views on these issues.

- Termination of pregnancy.
- Whether to have sex with the person you are currently in a relationship with.
- What to spend your money on.
- Suicide.

As this is a personal reflection, there is no outline answer at the end of the chapter.

Whether you identified your views as being moulded by your family, religion or rational thought, as you saw in Chapter 3, how our families are organised and the value we attach to rationality is influenced by our culture. In Chapter 3 we identified the pervading hegemony in the UK as a mix of paternalism, technologism and capitalism. In the UK our government is built on democracy. This, along with pervading hegemony, provides the environment to support two philosophical approaches that underpin decision-making when an ethical dilemma is raised: **paternalism** and **utilitarianism**. Under the paternalism approach a more powerful organisation or person takes control over another and states what is in the best interests of the other organisation or person. An example could be the ban on smoking in public places in England in 2006. The government was being paternalistic in taking away public choice in order to facilitate their health – their best interests. Utilitarianism is the approach of promoting the most happiness: so when a decision needs to be taken, the best course of action is the one that makes the most people happy. For example, a person enjoys playing their trumpet, but this disturbs their neighbours; using utilitarianism to decide what to do about it, the environment agency or landlord would endeavour to stop the person from playing their trumpet in that environment. While these approaches offer some understanding of decision-making and some guidance, they can be inadequate for making ethical decisions in health care.

You may have noticed that the terms **moral** and **ethical** have been used interchangeably. The distinction between moral and ethical is not clear and becomes even less clear when we acknowledge that ethics is defined as the study of morals. *'Morals' comes from the Latin moralis meaning custom, manner or law and 'ethics' comes from the Greek ethikos meaning custom or usage* (Docherty, 2011, pp67–68). Within nursing we tend to use the concept of morality for personal decisions on behaviours and attitudes, and the term ethics when we make professional decisions on behaviours or attitudes. Both are influenced by our pervading culture, and for many their moral stance reflects their religious beliefs.

> *Ethical care refers to good practice based on ethical values such as honesty, openness and trust.*
> (Brannelly, 2008, p244)

Biomedical ethical principles

Within health care the most widely accepted principles used to guide ethical decision-making are the biomedical ethics or principles set out by Beauchamp and Childress (2001). These principles are: **autonomy**, **justice**, **non-maleficence** and **beneficence**.

Autonomy comes from the Greek words *autos* (self) and *nomo* (law or rule); it therefore means self-rule or self-law. The ethical principle of autonomy refers to a person's ability to control their own life and make their own independent choices. Self-determination – control over one's environment – is important for maintaining a sense of self – identity, esteem and personhood. The saying that a person is a *law unto themselves* relates to autonomy in that the person is choosing to do what they wish without consideration for others. Autonomy is highly valued in our individualist society, and, as we have seen, it is important in person-centred humanised care. This saying can also, though, help us recognise that a person exhibiting autonomy without regard for others can create problems.

Justice comes from the Latin word *iustitia* (righteousness, equity) and has had a number of definitions, including lawful acts, fairness, equality and giving what is due. The dictionary definitions cover different types of justice: distributive, procedural, restorative and retributive. Distributive justice is about equity and fairness in what a person receives (economic justice). For example, if a nurse receives a letter of commendation from their manager for staying late to care for a distressed patient, so should another nurse for the same behaviour; it is her fair share. Procedural justice is about the decision-making process being seen as fair; this is fair play. Restorative justice tends to be about distribution or processes being considered unfair. In these situations the person seeks restoration. For example, one nurse is given the opportunity to attend a study day but another is not; the second nurse may seek restoration by asking to attend the next study day. Retributive justice is about a person seeking revenge for a behaviour that has caused them harm. This usually involves more than restoration; in this case, the person asks for the other person to experience at least the same level of discomfort. The ethical principles of justice focused on in health care are usually distributive and procedural justice: fair share and fair play.

Non-maleficence comes from the Latin words *non* (not, no) *mal* (bad) and *facere* (to do); 'do no bad' occurs when the person following this principle does not do or think things that could cause harm. This principle may be explored when, for example, a nurse is faced with providing a medical treatment that may make the person uncomfortable at the moment but is necessary for their long-term well-being.

The principle of *beneficence* comes from the Latin words *bene* (good) and *facere* (to do); 'do good' can simply be identified as doing good in thoughts, actions or attitudes. The bottom line for health care professionals, including nurses, is: if you cannot do anything else, 'do no harm'.

As you will know from your clinical practice, it is not easy to uphold all of these principles at the same time. Consider the case study of Brian Williams and his partner. How could the ethical principles guide his actions and your support of him?

Case study: Brian Williams

Brian lives in his own home with his partner, and he has Lewy body dementia. He frequently has disturbed sleep and at times has become quite distressed by seeing large dogs in his bedroom. More recently after he has been disturbed he has taken himself out of the house and walked around the village in his pyjamas until found – usually by his partner but one time by the police. This has led to his partner being frightened to go to sleep. Brian's partner is considering fitting locks to the bedroom door so that Brian cannot open it and wander off at night.

Activity 8.3   *Critical thinking*

What ethical issues may there be with locking Brian into his bedroom?

An outline answer is given at the end of the chapter.

Activity 8.3 helps you explore the ethical implications of removing Brian's liberty, and as a nurse you should work with Brian and his partner to make care decisions that uphold the ethical principles and Brian's human rights. Chapter 7 explored some of the care options open to you.

While the biomedical ethical principles are recognised as useful in clinical decision-making, these are not always felt to be the most useful in nursing care. Brannelly (2008) discusses the ethical principles within care that she found useful to understand the experiences of decision making in dementia care. The four principles that, she felt, facilitate good practice in a postmodern society were attentiveness, responsibility, competence and responsiveness. These principles could also be used in other areas of care.

Attentiveness refers to the nurse listening to or paying attention to the needs of the person with dementia. It is about putting the nurse's attitudes, beliefs and desires on one side and responding to the needs and desires of the person. *Responsibility* indicates the obligations the nurse has to respond to the needs and desires of the person once they have attended to and heard them. Once the nurse has recognised the need they should not then ignore that need.

It is already clear from the NMC code of conduct (2011) that nurses need to maintain and develop their competencies and skills, and not provide care where they do not have the appropriate knowledge and skills, but the principle of *competence* raised here as an ethic is wider than this. This ethic also involves the accessing and managing of resources to provide good care. If good care is not provided then competence is not achieved. *Responsiveness* refers to care as being a two-way communication: only the care receiver can inform us that the care received was good, so the nurse needs to respond to the cues given by the person, to adapt and change care when necessary.

This can be condensed to *What does the person receiving care want or need?* Once the nurse has established this they have the responsibility to provide it; only the person receiving care can judge the nurse's competence in providing care. The main principles here are the acceptance that each person is unique and the centrality of the person with dementia. The ethical principles discussed by Brannelly (2008) can be seen as relevant and important in caring for people with dementia in a humanised way. There are other ethical frameworks within dementia care and, like this one, they offer a process as well as underlying principles.

The ethical framework for dementia care described by the Nuffield Council for Bioethics (2009) offers nurses an opportunity for exploring the care given and a method for making evidence-based ethical decisions. This framework has six components.

- *Case-based approach* – this provides a three-stage process: identify the facts; apply ethical principles; seek differences and similarities with other cases to guide decision-making.
- *Beliefs about dementia* – this framework provides the belief that dementia is a brain disorder that is harmful to the person.
- *Belief about quality of life in dementia* – a person with dementia can still gain quality of life.
- *Importance of promoting the interests of the person with dementia and their carers* – promotion of autonomy and well-being of both the person and their carer is important as their experiences are intertwined, so a lack of well-being in the one has a negative impact on the other. Autonomy facilitates the person's sense of themselves and their ability to express what is important to them whether they have dementia or are the carer.
- *Requirement to work collaboratively* – as nurses, we need to recognise the uniqueness of the person but also to acknowledge our interdependence and responsibility to support them. We therefore need to work collaboratively with the person and their carers.
- *Acknowledgement of personhood, identity and value* – if a person has dementia, it should not affect their value or worth. They should be respected for the unique person they are, regardless of the severity of the disease.

As with Brannelly (2008), the Nuffield framework offers a process of gathering evidence and applying it and the principle of the person as unique, but it also offers a wider perspective. This includes respect for the person with dementia and their carers, an acknowledgement of the disorder, and the belief that quality of life is still achievable.

One of the biggest ethical and legal dilemmas in dementia care is consent to treatment when a person's cognitive ability is deteriorating, and it is consent that we will look at next.

Consent

The code: standards of conduct, performance and ethics for nurses and midwives (NMC, 2011) clearly states:

13. *You must ensure that you gain consent before you begin any treatment or care.*
14. *You must respect and support people's right to accept or decline treatment and care.*
15. *You must uphold people's rights to be fully involved in decisions about their care.*

As you can see, as nurses we need to explain what the care intervention is, gain the person's consent to our providing this care and accept their decision if they choose not to receive it.

Activity 8.4   *Critical thinking*

Make a list of all the activities that could be involved in caring for a person with dementia.

Some examples are given at the end of the chapter.

The majority of nursing activities could be considered treatment or care, so it is important that consent is sought with every activity we undertake with or to another person in our nursing role. In the following case study, despite Peter's attempts to gain informed consent, he did not achieve it. If a person you are caring for refuses care or treatment, how might you respond?

Case study: Peter

Peter is a student nurse; he has been placed on a medical ward and as part of his learning he is assisting the registered nurse to administer medication. When he reaches Mrs Little he greets her and informs her that he is a student nurse and is helping the registered nurse with the medication. He tells her what is on her prescription chart and explains that it is the same medication that she had at the same time yesterday. Peter then, under the supervision of the registered nurse, puts Mrs Little's medication in a pot and attempts to put the pot in her hand. Mrs Little shouts at Peter: I am not going to take that poison.

Activity 8.5   *Critical thinking*

Why do you think Mrs Little might have refused the medication and suggested it was poison?

There is an outline answer at the end of the chapter.

There are many reasons why Mrs Little may have refused her medication, but whatever the reason, Peter should continue to behave respectfully towards her. He could seek to find out why she was refusing the medication, as she may just have misheard what he has said, which could quickly be addressed. If she did not want the medication given to her by him because he was male or a student, her wishes need to be taken into account when her care is provided. If Mrs Little is unable to articulate why she says the medication is poisoned, further assessment of her health may need exploring, such as whether she has the ability to understand the treatment and whether she has a mental health problem.

If after assessment by the interprofessional team and her family it is decided Mrs Little does not have the capacity to make the decision or that her mental health problem is interfering with her ability to make the decision, there are specific laws to guide nurses how to deal with these situations. If she is unable to make decisions due to her inability to understand the information, she can be cared for under the Mental Capacity Act and if she has a significant mental health problem that is interfering with her ability to make decisions, she can be cared for under the Mental Health Act. Both of these laws will be explored later in this chapter.

The legal context

Ethics can guide the interpretation of law but cannot justify the breaking of law. To return to the example given in the introduction, some nurses may believe it is cruel or immoral to keep someone alive when their death is imminent and they are in pain. Ethically, they might believe it is right to assist in their death. To assist in another person's death is illegal and to undertake this act could lead to prosecution for manslaughter or murder. The ethical belief of the person cannot justify breaking the law.

All complex societies need laws to establish what is unacceptable behaviour for that society. We have two types of law in the UK.

• Common law.
• Statutory law.

Common law is created by the exploration of cases; it is therefore based on case law or precedent. An example of this is **negligence**. The law in this area has developed over a fairly short period of time. Negligence occurs where there is harm to a person through the lack of appropriate care by, for example, a nurse. Whether a nurse is found guilty of negligence will depend on previous cases where negligence has been found to have occurred. If the nurse is found guilty in a particular case, it will become part of case law or common law. As you can see, if each case builds on the previous cases, what is considered to be negligence could change fairly quickly.

Common law is more adaptable than statutory law, reflecting changes within society; statutory law needs to go through a number of stages to become a statute or act of law. Acts of law are generated through pressure groups, EU directives, government established policy groups and experts in the field. Revisions to the England and Wales Mental Health Act in 2007, for example, are shown in Figure 8.1.

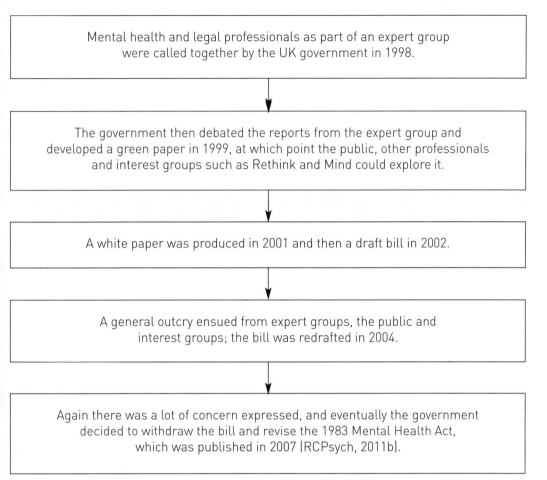

Figure 8.1: Revisions to the England and Wales Mental Health Act

Human Rights Act

The Human Rights Act of 1998 came into force in the UK in 2000. This was part of European law that went through the statutory processes in the UK and has now become part of UK law. The rights set out in this act are:

- the right to life;
- freedom from torture and inhumane or degrading treatment;
- right to liberty and security;
- freedom from slavery and forced labour;
- right to a fair trial;
- no punishment without law;
- respect for private life, home and correspondence;
- freedom of thought, belief and religion;
- freedom of expression;
- freedom of assembly and association;
- right to marry and start a family;

- protection from discrimination;
- right to peaceful enjoyment of your property;
- right to education;
- right to participate in free elections.

While all these rights appear acceptable and just, we can see that there are a number of issues that relate to nursing care. For example, do we always provide space for freedom of expression? Protection from discrimination? The right to liberty? We could be found guilty of breaking the human rights law if we do not uphold these rights.

Activity 8.6   *Critical thinking*

Can you think of any occasions where it is acceptable to breach a person's human rights?

An outline answer is given at the end of the chapter.

There are laws that take precedence over the Human Rights Act as laid out here, but they are and should be interpreted as correlating with the principles of human rights law. Two of these laws are the Mental Capacity Act and the Mental Health Act.

Mental Capacity Act

The Mental Capacity Act (MCA) was first published in 2005 but came into force in 2007 as part of the revision to the Mental Health Act (MHA), but these acts only apply in England and Wales. In Scotland there is the Adults with Incapacity Act (2000), and in Northern Ireland mental health and capacity are under review with a new law expected to be enacted in 2013.

The main principles of the Act are (Docherty, 2011, p88):

- a presumption of capacity;
- individuals being supported to make their own decisions;
- acceptance that people make unwise decisions;
- if decisions need to be made for others, they are in their best interests;
- if decisions need to be made for others, they are the least restrictive ones.

The initial assumption is that the person has the capacity to make their own decisions unless they have been assessed, at this time, not to have capacity. The Act is accompanied by a detailed code of practice, which was published in 2007, and this is the basis for the rest of this section.

To make an assessment of incapacity the person will not be able to:

- understand the information relevant to the decision;
- retain information for long enough periods to make a decision on it;
- use the information in their decision-making;
- communicate their decision.
  (MCA, 2005, section 3(1))

All of these areas may be problematic for a person with dementia, but the Act clearly supports the principles of person-centred care in that initial assumptions need to be that the person has capacity. It is only when the person has been assessed as not having capacity to make a judgement 'at this time' that decisions can be made on their behalf in their best interest. The term 'at this time' was a deliberate inclusion, as a person may have fluctuating capacity and be able to make some decisions but not others, given the above criteria.

Best interests

If decisions are to be made for the person when they have been assessed as lacking capacity, these must be undertaken in the person's **best interest** and be the **least restrictive**.

Assessing best interest is usually conducted within the multi-disciplinary team, but the responsible medical officer usually signs the form. The following need consideration.

- Whether the person may regain capacity.
- Whether the person can participate in decision-making.
- The fact that any desire to bring about the death of the person should not influence the decision.
- The person's past and present wishes or feelings.
- Any written statement made previously by the person.
- The beliefs and values that would have influenced the person's decision.
- Other relevant factors.
  (Hodge, 2008)

The Act also offers guidance on who could help the decision-maker's identification of best interest.

- Anyone named to be consulted for decisions in respect of this person.
- The carer or others interested in the person's welfare.
- The donee of any Lasting Power of Attorney (this will be discussed later in this section).
- Any deputy appointed by the court.
  (Hodge, 2008, p269)

The case study of Bethany Milner offers an example of implementing best interests.

Case study: Bethany Milner

*Bethany is a patient on a medical ward, and she has been there for four weeks. She was admitted to the ward after being found unconscious in the local town but has been physically fit for discharge for a couple of weeks. Bethany has a diagnosis of Alzheimer's dementia and had been found lost and confused by the police before. She lives in her family home where she is supported by a comprehensive care package, but this is provided by a number of carers. Her children, who are **donees of a lasting power of attorney**, live some distance away. A case review has been organised by the gerontologist responsible for her care. Bethany's children, the care providers, a nurse and an occupational therapist from the ward all attend the review. In the previous*

continued . . .

> *review of Bethany's case at the memory clinic it was decided that she no longer had capacity to make decisions. Her children and the nurses knew Bethany would like to live in her own home if this was at all possible, so the current package, as the least restrictive option, was set up. For the current review Bethany does not appear to understand what is being asked of her when her opinion is sought. It is decided that Bethany still does not have capacity to make her own decisions and that she is unlikely to regain capacity. It is decided that in her best interests Bethany should be accommodated in a nursing home.*

Other elements of the Act not mentioned above are:

- advance decision-making; advance directives;
- court of protection;
- independent mental capacity advocates;
- negligence made a criminal act when involving people without capacity;
- refers to people over 16;
- lasting power of attorney.

The elements 'negligence made a criminal act' and 'refers to people over 16' are quite clear, but the other components need further clarification.

Advance decision-making

For many years there has been discussion about 'living wills', but there was no obligation that when a person was unable to make their own decisions these would influence the person's care. The Mental Capacity Act in section 24 provides a legal basis for a person to make decisions while they have capacity about future treatment if they should become incapacitated. This section only addresses legal issues of consent, though, so advance directives (advance decision-making) relate to treatments that the person would refuse if they still had mental capacity.

Despite this, as seen above, when making decisions in the person's best interest, any indication of what the person would have wished should be taken into account. A bigger problem with advance decision-making is that it is impossible for anyone to predict exactly what is going to happen and all the possible options related to the situation. There will always be the need for those acting in the best interest of the person to interpret what would be wished in a specific circumstance.

Having an early diagnosis of dementia is particularly important if the person has strong beliefs about how they should be treated towards the end of their life. If they have the diagnosis, they can make advance decisions while they have capacity with the knowledge available on the progression of the disease and treatment choices.

Independent mental capacity advocates (IMCA)

The aim of the IMCA service is to provide independent safeguards for people who lack capacity to make certain important decisions, and at the time such decisions need to be made, have no one else (other than paid staff) to support or represent them or be consulted.
(MCA, 2007, p178)

Section 35–41 of the Mental Capacity Act (MCA, 2005) deals with independent mental capacity advocates. Section 36 (2) indicates the role of the IMCA is to:

- provide support to the person they are representing so that the person may participate as fully as possible in any relevant decision;
- obtain and evaluate relevant information;
- ascertain what the person's wishes and feelings would be, and the beliefs and values that would be likely to influence them;
- ascertain what alternatives are available;
- obtain a further medical opinion where treatment is proposed and they think it is necessary.

The Act states that the appropriate authority should ensure IMCAs are available to those that need them. For England, this is the Secretary of State and for Wales it is the Welsh Assembly.

Lasting power of attorney

Within the Mental Capacity Act (MCA, 2005) there is provision for a role of lasting power of attorney (LPA), which replaces the enduring power of attorney that preceded the MCA. Lasting power of attorney is where the person, legally known as a donor, while they still have capacity, identifies a person or persons to manage on their behalf their legal, financial and health matters. For an LPA to make decisions on the person's behalf when they have lost capacity, they need to be registered with the Office of the Public Guardian (OPG) while the person still has capacity.

The donor can make an LPA for personal welfare or property and financial affairs. To do this the donor must have a certificate that states they currently have capacity to make the decision and to fill in the appropriate forms from the OPG. To become registered as an attorney, the person must be over 18 and not bankrupt. The OPG then deals with any issues arising, such as complaints about the LPA.

The court of protection

The court of protection has wide-ranging powers that are similar to that of the High Court in England and Wales. It has the authority to:

- make decisions on a person's mental capacity;
- make decisions on financial or welfare matters for people who lack capacity;
- decide whether a lasting power of attorney is legal;
- remove LPAs who do not fulfil their duties;
- listen to objections to the registration of LPAs.

If a person who lacks capacity does not have an LPA, the court of protection can appoint someone to make decisions for them; this person is referred to as a **deputy**. Deputies are usually close friends or family, but a professional such as a solicitor could also be appointed as a deputy and they need to act in accordance with the MCA seeking the person's best interests using the least restrictive approach.

Although the Mental Capacity Act can provide protection and support for a person with dementia who lacks capacity, dementia is defined as a mental disorder under the Mental Health Act and so people with dementia could have their care managed under this piece of legislation. When the Mental Health Act is enacted, it does not mean the person lacks capacity to make decisions. Many people who have a mental disorder and are sectioned under the Mental Health Act retain the capacity to make most of their own decisions; it is only decisions relevant to their mental disorder that are being legislated for in this Act.

Mental Health Act

As identified in a previous section, the Mental Health Act (MHA) for England and Wales that is in operation now was written in 1983 but has gone through a few changes in the intervening years, the most recent published in 2007. The Mental Health (Care and Treatment) (Scotland) Act (2003) came into effect in 2005, and in Northern Ireland the Mental Health Act 1986 is under review, with the expectation of a joint Mental Health and Mental Capacity Bill being enacted in 2013. Regardless of which Act you consider, the components of a Mental Health Act are going to provide legislation on the following.

- What constitutes a mental disorder/mental illness in relation to the Act; who the Act refers to or what its terms of reference are.
- When the person with a mental disorder can have their liberty restricted.
- When the person can be given treatment against their will.
- What the person's rights are related to these issues.
- The safeguards that are in place to ensure the Act is not misused.

The case study of Elsie Robinson may help you understand the process of enacting the Mental Health Act in England and Wales (1983/2007).

Case study: Elsie Robinson

Elsie was diagnosed with Lewy body dementia four years ago and has recently been living in a residential care home. Elsie's behaviour has become increasingly erratic and at times she has appeared to be looking into space and speaking to people who are not in the room. This has increased, and it seems that whatever Elsie is hearing it is very unpleasant as she shouts and swears in response. The shouting and screaming is particularly a problem at night, disturbing the other residents and leading to Elsie hitting the night staff when they try to encourage calm. If the carers try to comfort her, she hits out at them even during the day. The carers feel it is becoming impossible to offer her personal care due what they feel is unpredictable aggression.

*Elsie is visited by her GP who refers her to the older persons' community mental health team. She is assessed by a nurse and a psychiatrist but she refuses to accept any of the interventions they offer or any medication. She also refuses an admission to a mental health assessment ward so that an assessment of her needs can be made. The psychiatrist and nurse feel Elsie is a risk to herself and others, so they instigate an MHA assessment. An **approved mental health practitioner (AMHP)** is called to assess Elsie. They feel that Elsie needs to be assessed in an in-patient setting. The AMHP completes an application for detention in a psychiatric*

continued . . .

> *hospital under Section 2 of the Mental Health Act, and two doctors – one who knows Elsie (her GP) and one*
> *approved under section 12 of the MHA (the psychiatrist) – make formal recommendations for the application*
> *of the section.*
>
> *Once the paperwork is completed, Elsie is escorted to the mental health unit by the ambulance crew and a carer*
> *from the home.*

In the case study of Elsie we can see that Section 2 of the MHA was the one chosen to provide appropriate care for her. There a few key sections of the MHA that are particularly relevant to people with dementia, and these are Section 2, Section 3, Section 4, Sections 5 (2) and 5 (4), Section 132 and Section 136. These are all briefly outlined in Table 8.1.

Section of MHA	Duration	Who can implement it	Purpose
2	28 days	Needs: 1 AMHP application and 2 Medical recommendations (one who knows the person and one approved under section 12)	Assessment
3	6 months	Needs: 1 AMHP application and 2 Medical recommendations (one who knows the person and one approved under section 12)	Treatment
4	72 hours	Needs: 1 AMHP application and 1 Medical recommendation	Emergency assessment
5 (2)	72 hours	1 doctor but person needs to be in hospital already	Doctor's holding power
5 (4)	6 hours	1 registered mental health nurse but person must be in hospital already	Nurse's holding power
132		Mental health professional, usually a nurse	Obligation to inform person of their rights under the MHA
136	72 hours	Police officer	Removal from a public place to a place of safety

Table 8.1: Overview of common MHA sections

A person can be taken to a mental health unit against their will under sections 2, 3, 4 and 136 of the MHA. There are other sections that would allow a person to be taken to a mental health unit, but they are not particularly relevant to people with dementia. The MHA also has provision for giving people psychiatric treatment against their will, but as with any other area of health care it is always best to work with people in a humanised manner, so it is only a small minority of people with a mental disorder who are treated under the MHA.

You can see that people can legally be deprived of their liberty if they fulfil the criteria to be treated under a section of the MHA ('sectioned'). Some people necessarily have their freedom restricted without being detained through the MHA, and there are safeguards put in place to protect people in this position.

Deprivation of liberty

Deprivation of liberty does not have a refined definition as there are a wide number of actions that fulfil this term. Undertake Activity 8.7 to explore what you might identify as an adequate definition.

Activity 8.7   *Critical thinking*

Which of the situations below do you think constitute a deprivation of liberty?

- A person standing in your way so you cannot leave a room.
- The door lock being so complicated you cannot work out how to get out.
- The door being locked and you do not have a key.
- Being told you have to wait before you can have a drink.
- Being refused a meal.
- Having tablets hidden in your food.
- Not being allowed to go for a walk with friends.
- Having a radio station you do not like playing continuously.
- Being restrained, held down.

There is an outline answer at the end of the chapter.

As you should have noticed, there are numerous occasions where a person could be considered to have their liberty removed. A broad definition of it could be the restriction of freedom or choice. Under the Mental Capacity Act there is a provision for the deprivation of liberty but this can only legally occur under the Act if a person is deprived of their liberty in order to do a vital act or treatment to sustain life (MCA, 2005). Alongside this is the provision of deprivation of liberty safeguards (DOLS); these safeguards are for people who lack capacity but are not treated under the Mental Health Act and therefore not protected by the safeguards associated with it.

Safeguarding

There have been a number of government documents developed to safeguard vulnerable people, which have been necessary because some adults have been abused both in the home setting and in institutional care settings. In 2000 the Department of Health published the *No secrets* document (DH, 2000) in recognition that abuse of adults was a hidden and secret activity. This has been followed up with developments to the Mental Health Act and Mental Capacity Act to protect the vulnerable. In 2011 the government provided further guidance in the form of the *Safeguarding adults* document (DH, 2011c). In this document six principles were laid down.

- Empowerment – ensuring patient-centred care, the person is at the centre being enabled to make choices.
- Protection – ensuring no harm is done to the person.
- Prevention – managing the situation so that protection is not needed.
- Proportionality – ensuring any action is in proportion to the need; least restrictive intervention.
- Partnership – working collaboratively with the person.
- Accountability – ensuring there is a clear understanding of actions taken and why.

Within the Mental Capacity Act there are specific documents safeguarding those who lack capacity to ensure that liberty is deprived only when it is absolutely necessary (DH, 2009). This policy is not to enforce treatment; it is more about people who are not able to express an opinion or consent to treatment. The case study of Eric Robins will give you an example of how the MCA provides a process to ensure that the rights of a person with dementia are safeguarded.

Case study: Eric Robins

Eric has been found standing in the middle of the road, and this has led the nursing staff in the nursing home to become concerned for his safety. Eric has Alzheimer's dementia and his condition has slowly deteriorated throughout his stay. The nurses have used distraction to encourage him to stay in the home unless someone is able to escort him on his walks. The nurses believe he lacks mental capacity to make the decisions related to his personal safety. They would like to introduce a care plan to address their perception of Eric's needs, which would restrict his going for a walk unless there is a member of staff to escort him. The matron is concerned that without a decision on Eric's mental capacity, ongoing restriction of his liberty would be unlawful. As Eric has no family or close friends, the matron seeks advice under the deprivation of liberty safeguards from the supervisory body (the local NHS Trust). They arrange for two assessors to check the care being given to Eric. The one assessor is identified as the 'best interests' assessor and the other a mental health assessor. It is decided that in this situation Eric is unable to assess the risks involved in his behaviour, and that he therefore lacks mental capacity. To deprive him of the liberty to take himself alone for walks is deemed in his best interests as long as he is facilitated in going for a walk with a member of staff as part of his planned care. The assessors request that an independent mental capacity advocate is appointed to support the ongoing assessment of Eric's mental capacity and to seek his best interests.

Alongside government legislation such as the MCA and the 2011 safeguarding document there are other mechanisms to protect vulnerable people. All nurses are required to complete a criminal records bureau (CRB) assessment prior to starting their degree programmes and throughout their career. The NMC recognises the crucial importance of safeguarding. They have developed ways to protect the public through statutory requirements of nurses such as the code of conduct, fitness to practice boards and whistle-blowing expectations. They also provide guidelines on managing, safeguarding and support that can be accessed on their safeguarding hub (see Useful websites at the end of the chapter).

Chapter summary

This chapter has briefly explored ethical decision-making in nursing people with dementia and the legal framework within which nurses need to work. The biomedical ethical principles of Beauchamp and Childress (autonomy, justice, non-maleficence and beneficence) are those most frequently used in health care, but there are other ethical frameworks that can support ethical decision-making in dementia care nursing. Those considered here were those discussed by Brannelly (2008) – attention, responsibility, competence and responsiveness – and the six Nuffield bioethics. While it is important that nurses make ethically appropriate decisions, ethical decisions need to made within the law.

Acts of law that are particularly relevant to dementia care nursing are the Human Rights Act, Mental Capacity Act and the Mental Health Act. The MCA and MHA explored in this chapter are those relating to England and Wales, as Scotland and Northern Ireland have different laws addressing capacity and mental health. The chapter ended with a brief consideration of deprivation of liberty and safeguards for vulnerable people such as those with dementia. The government and our professional body, the NMC, both have requirements of nurses and guidance to support us to safeguard vulnerable people.

Activities: brief outline answers

Activity 8.3: Critical thinking (page 147)

There are numerous problems with locking Brian into his bedroom; they can be separated into safety, legal and moral/ethical categories.

*   Safety – if there was a fire, Brian would not be able to escape.
*   Legal – it is illegal to imprison another person without a section of the law being placed upon them.
*   Moral/ethical – this will take away Brian's autonomy, reduce his self-esteem and raise his anxieties and fears. It could be seen as maleficent (doing harm) for the reasons already stated and unjust, given that it is illegal and that other people with dementia will not be locked in a room.

Activity 8.4: Critical thinking (page 149)

Some examples could be:

*   administering medication;
*   feeding;

- washing/dressing;
- taking the person to the toilet;
- taking stitches out;
- dressing a wound;
- taking a blood pressure reading.

Activity 8.5: Critical thinking (page 149)

It is difficult to know why Mrs Little refused her medication and said it was poisoned without asking her, but there are a number of possible reasons.

- She did not trust the student.
- She does not like men.
- Yesterday's medication made her feel unwell.
- She believes people are trying the poison her.
- She misheard or misunderstood what had been said to her.
- She misperceived what was happening.

Activity 8.6: Critical thinking (page 152)

It may be considered acceptable to remove a person's liberty if it is to protect them from harm: see the section of deprivation of liberty.

Decisions are made about who should receive an organ transplant based on a number of factors that could be considered discriminatory, such as age and health status.

If a person is expressing opinions that offend others or incite violence, they may be in contravention of another law, and the judicial system will need to make a decision as to which takes precedence.

Activity 8.7: Critical thinking (page 158)

All of these actions could constitute a deprivation of liberty.

Further reading

Hughs, J and Baldwin, C (2006) *Ethical issues in dementia care: making difficult decisions.* London: Jessica Kingsley Publishers.

This short book offers an easy-to-read approach to explain ethics in dementia care and how difficult ethical decisions can be made.

Useful websites

www.legislation.gov.uk/ukpga/2005/9/contents

This government website offers the opportunity to explore the Mental Capacity Act in detail along with an overview of it.

www.legislation.gov.uk/ukpga/2007/12/contents

This government website allows you to explore the various elements of the Mental Health Act as well as giving an overview of its provision.

www.nmc-uk.org/Nurses-and-midwives/safeguarding

On this NMC hub you can access the NMC guidance for safeguarding as well as other practitioners' good practice and a training resource.

Glossary

abuse   to misuse; to treat someone badly

accommodation   a concept within Piaget's cognitive developmental theory meaning the development of a new schema when new information makes an old schema obsolete.

acute confusional state   acute: of short duration; a sudden or of short duration state of being confused or disorientated about time, place or person.

ageism   a type of discrimination based on the person's age – usually related to older age but can be used for younger ages too.

agency   a person's ability to act for themselves; to undertake an action based on their free will.

agnosia   the absence (a) of the ability to recognise or identify objects.

antidepressants   a group of medications primarily used to treat depression. There are different pharmacological categories, including tricyclics, specific serotonin reuptake inhibitors and monoamine oxidase inhibitors.

approved mental health practitioner (AMHP)   a mental health practitioner such as a social worker, mental health nurse or occupational therapist who has undertaken a further qualification to become 'approved' to conduct mental health assessments in order to complete an application for a person to be detained under the Mental Health Act.

apraxia   the absence (a) of the ability to control bodily actions (movements).

assimilation   a concept within Piaget's cognitive developmental theory, meaning the incorporation of new information into an existing schema; the information is assimilated.

atrial fibrillation   a cardiac dysrhythmia, i.e. the heart is not maintaining its usual rhythm. This particular dysrhythmia is where the atria (the upper chambers of the heart) are not beating properly – they are fibrillating (flickering).

attitudes   the emotional, cognitive and behavioural response to underlying beliefs and values of the person.

auditory   pertaining to the perception of hearing.

autonomy   making one's own choices or decisions.

beneficence   doing good.

best interest   to do something or make a decision on someone else's behalf in order to facilitate what they would have done, if able, to promote their own health or well-being.

celebration   one of the positive person work interventions identified by Kitwood, where nurses provide the opportunity for the person to recognise and express a joy about something with other people.

centring   the disregarding of personal attitudes and values to focus on the person and their concerns; to put the person at the centre. This can be done by controlling one's breathing and paying attention to the person.

cerebral cortex   the main, biggest, part of the brain and has two parts.

cerebral hypoxia   cerebral: brain; hypoxia: a lack of oxygen. The brain is receiving too little oxygen.

cognitively challenged   usually refers to a person who is struggling to process their thoughts.

commodification   the treatment of something or someone as a commodity that can be bought and sold.

concept   an idea or collection of ideas that work together as a whole idea/thought/entity.

confabulated/confabulation   to make up a story/explanation; this term is usually associated with mental disorder, particularly Korsakov's syndrome.

constructs   the elements or parts of a theory.

continuum   a continuing string of items/ideas/thoughts where those next to each other are difficult to distinguish apart but each end of the string are opposing – the opposite of each other.

correlation   the finding that different things occur in the same situation. A statistical approach might seek correlations between certain behaviours, thoughts or attitudes, but if a correlation is found, it does not mean that the one caused the other to happen – only that they occurred together.

cortical encephalopathy   cortical: relates to the brain; encephalopathy: an abnormal structure or function of brain tissue. This condition is usually found in degenerative diseases. A disease of the outer part of the brain.

crystallised intelligence   experientially dependent; it relates to the person's experiences and includes abilities such as knowledge for general information and verbal comprehension.

cyanosis   literally, the blue disease; this relates to a blueish colour to the skin due to lack of oxygen in the blood usually seen first in lips and nail beds.

deductive reasoning   reasoning or decision-making using rational and logical thought processes; working through a problem one step at a time.

deputy   in the context of the Mental Capacity Act someone appointed by the court of protection to make decisions for the person lacking capacity, ensuring the decisions are the least restrictive and in the person's best interests.

differential diagnosis   a different diagnosis; whether an alternative assessment of the person's problems can be made.

discrimination   where decisions on how to respond to a person are made on the basis of a stereotype and the action has negative consequences for the person.

donees of a lasting power of attorney   under the Mental Capacity Act the persons who are legally appointed by the donor to make decisions for them when or if they lose capacity.

dynamic   being in a state of always changing, moving or developing.

dysphasia/aphasia   difficulty (dys) or absence (a) of speech.

ego   I; the person's sense of themselves. In psychodynamic theory it is the part of the self that balances the needs and desires of the id against the social and moral codes of the superego.

electrocardiogram   a machine that measures the electrical activity of the heart.

embodiment   a recognition that the social, psychological and spiritual person exists within a physical body, therefore all elements of the person need consideration in care situations.

episodic memory   the ability to recall specific situations; to remember separate episodes.

ethical   decisions about what professional behaviour or attitudes are right or wrong.

ethology   the study of animal behaviour and how it occurs in the natural environment.

explicitly   clearly and fully defined, leaving nothing to be assumed or implied.

familial   pertaining to the family, for example genetic disorders.

fibrils   small fibres. Amyloidal fibrils: small fibres made up of insoluble proteins that impact on the functioning of brain cells in dementia.

fluid intelligence   physiologically dependent; it relates to the body's ability and involves activities such as perceptual speed and visual organisation.

functional   able to fulfil its role; the body is working as it should.

hallucination   the perception of something that is not present; can occur in all of the senses but is most commonly visual (sight) or auditory (hearing).

hegemony   the predominance of one social class or ideology over others.

hippocampus   a part of the limbic system in the brain lying at the bottom of the lateral ventricles and involved in memory and emotions.

hyperactive   over active.

hypertension   high blood pressure.

hypoactive   under active.

iatrogenic   illness or disease due to medical intervention.

id   according to psychodynamic theory, the innate part of the personality that demands to have its needs/desires addressed immediately.

ideology   a set of beliefs or a worldview; a system of abstract views that address the social and aspirational needs of a group.

impaired higher cortical functioning   the reduced ability of the brain, particularly the frontal lobes, to undertake activities such as reasoning and problem solving.

implicitly   implied, not stated clearly and unambiguously.

insiderness   a term used within the model of care developed by Todres et al. (2009), which indicates that carers should recognise/understand what the person is experiencing in their perceptual world.

insidious   of slow onset.

interdisciplinary   something that is done by two or more disciplines working together.

intuitive   where a decision is based on instinct rather than rational, logical, conscious reasoning.

justice   being fair.

least restrictive   where the fewest restrictions or limitations are placed on the person to facilitate the greatest amount of autonomy within the boundaries of the disease and resources.

Lewy bodies   concentric spheres made up of proteins.

lifeworld   the total experience of the person – their inner thoughts and feelings along with their social and interactional experiences.

linear process   a movement; a process that goes in one direction, one step after another.

linking behaviour   one behaviour that is associated or linked with another.

malignant social psychology (MSP)   a concept highlighted by Kitwood when exploring the care of people with dementia. He found that carers behaved in ways that reduced the person's self-concept and self-esteem without intending to, through using accepted cultural responses.

manifests   occurs, happens, appears.

mean   a number of meanings but in this context a type of average; a mathematical concept. There are three types of average: mode, median and mean. To establish a mean you need to add all the numbers up (e.g. $12 + 22 + 32 + 42 = 108$) and then divide by the number of numbers (4); this gives the mean average (27 in this example).

mental defence mechanisms   a concept identified by Freud. They are coping strategies used by people when in psychological difficulty; in the short term they can be helpful, but in the long term they reduce the person's ability to get on with their life in a healthy manner.

mirroring   the copying of the behaviour of one person by another.

mixed economy   an economy that utilises both public and private funds.

model   a proposed structure or way of organising actions.

moral   personal decisions about what behaviour or attitudes are right.

mortality   refers to death, the incidence or number of deaths.

multi-dimensional   more than one dimension; more than one way of viewing something.

multi-infarct   more than one infarct; more than one obstruction to the blood supply leading to the death of cells.

multiple higher cortical functions   many functions of the higher cortex: memory, thinking, orientation, comprehension, calculation, learning capacity, language and judgement.

myelinisation   the process of nerve cells being covered with myelin (made from cholesterol), which protects and speeds the nerve impulse.

myelopathy   damage to spinal cord.

negligence   not providing proper care, which could lead to harm to the person.

negotiate   to reach an agreement through discussion.

neural fibrillary tangles   small fibres that develop from within the neurone. They interfere with the normal functioning of the neurone.

neurochemical   relating to chemicals that are found in or affect the nervous system.

neuronal plasticity   the ability of nerves to adapt, develop and change.

neuropathological   diseases of neurones or the nervous system.

neuropathy   damage to nerves.

non-declarative memory   memory for how to do things that are difficult to declare or explain but easier to show, such as tying shoe laces or riding a bicycle.

non-maleficence   doing no harm.

opiates   drugs developed from opium, such as morphine; they have strong pain-killing functions.

organic   in the context of people, refers to an organ of the body; organic disease is a disease of a part of the body.

orthodoxy   behaving in the right way according to set rules usually related to a religious belief system.

ownness   from the philosophy of phenomenology, which influenced the development of the humanising care model by Todres et al. It means to be and belong to one's self.

paternalism   an ideology that promotes the acceptance of a 'father figure' or 'powerful other' such as the government who knows best and makes decisions on behalf of others without their explicit consent.

pathophysiology   changes in the body's structure or functioning due to disease.

perceptual world   the person's experience of the world through their senses; the person's interpretation of their senses.

personal journey   one of the elements of Todres et al.'s model of care referring to the individual nature of how a person progresses through life along with their understanding, desires and goals.

plaques   a number of different types of plaques can be found in the body. Most importantly for dementia are senile and atherosclerotic plaques. Senile plaques are a spherical group of amyloidal fibres in the brain and atherosclerotic plaques start from fatty deposits in the arteries.

polypharmacy   the use of a number of medicines at the same time.

positive person work   a person-centred approach to care developed by Kitwood to address the problem of malignant social psychology.

preferred sense   the sense the person prefers to use, probably the one that functions best. A person who struggles with their sight might prefer to listen to information.

prevalence   the number of people experiencing a certain condition at a given time.

procedural   in the context of memory, refers to the ability to remember how to do something.

proprioception   the perceptual information from the senses that allow the person to identify where parts of their body are.

psychopathology   pathology: disease or ill health; psyche: of the mind; disease of the mind.

relaxation   the experience of being at rest, free from tension or stress.

reminiscing   thinking about things that have already happened; thinking about the past.

rephrasing   saying what has already been said using different words.

response   an action occurring due to a stimulus.

risk factor   something that could cause harm.

role model   a person who acts out how things should or could be done for others to learn from.

schema theory   a cognitive theory that knowledge and information (memory) is stored in the brain in packets or collections, together with elements that link one schema to another.

self-actualisation   from the humanist approach, the experience of achieving one's potential, a peak experience. However, the person is not able to maintain this position and needs to start at the bottom of hierarchy again.

self-efficacy   the belief in our ability to achieve our goals.

self-esteem   the worth or value we attach to ourselves.

semantic memory   memory or recall related to knowledge and understanding.

sense of place   a concept in Todres et al.'s model of care that refers to a sense of belonging; the experience of being at home.

short-term memory   the ability to hold information for short periods of time to allow manipulation or use of it.

social exclusion   where people are rejected or their worth is not acknowledged by their community or society, usually due to gender, age, religion, race or disability.

spatiality   a concept from phenomenological philosophy that underpins Todres et al.'s model of care. It concerns a person's ability to understand their place in time and space; to understand their contextual situation both historically and in the present.

sporadic   occurs at irregular intervals without an identified cause.

stepwise   a progression of disease distinguished by a period of stability, then an acute step down to a reduced level of ability.

stereotypes   the application of certain characteristics to a group of people without reference to the individual differences between them.

stigmatise   to degrade a person due to a particular circumstance they find themselves in.

stimulus   something that arouses or motivates a person to action.

sub-cortical encephalopathy   an abnormal structure or function of brain tissue. Sub: under; cortical: brain, encephalopathy; this condition is usually found in degenerative diseases. It is therefore a disease of the inner part of the brain.

superego   according to psychodynamic theory, the part of the mind that has developed from the environment and is known as the conscience. It tries to force the person to comply with rules and behave morally.

synaptic growth   synapses or links between neurones are being made, which facilitate increased brain function.

syndrome   a group of signs or symptoms that when found in a collection are labelled together.

temporal lobe   lobe in the brain on either side of the head. The brain has two cerebral hemispheres – one on the left of the body and one on the right – and these are further divided into lobes. The frontal lobe is at the front of the head, the occipital lobe is at the back of the head, the parietal lobe is in between and the temporal lobe is on either side of the head.

temporality   a concept from the philosophy of phenomenology that means existing in time, a relationship with time.

timalation   an activity as part of positive person work established by Kitwood. It refers to the need to experience the world through all of the senses: through touch, smell, sound, sight and taste.

togetherness   a concept within the model of care by Todres et al. and refers to the need to experience the world with other people. This is also acknowledged by Kitwood.

trajectory   the expected progress or journey of a condition.

turgor   refers to the skin's ability to return to its usual shape; its elasticity. If a person is dehydrated, the skin will not have its usual turgor and take some time to return to its usual shape when pinched.

uniqueness   to be distinct or different from others; to be one of a kind.

utilitarianism   an ideology common in Western society that facilitates the 'greater good' when a moral or ethical decision is needed. The right choice is the one that achieves the most people being happy.

validating   acknowledging a person's perspective and recognising its importance for them.

variant   a type of something that differs from the usual.

vascular   pertaining to the blood vessels.

vicariously   occurring indirectly or through someone else.

visuospatial   refers to the visual perception of the relationship between objects: the distance between objects.

visual   relating to sight.

whole systems approach   an approach that looks at how all systems within a certain context work together, not focusing on individual ones – for example, with people, avoiding focusing on the biological system only.

References

Adams, S (2011) Up to three-quarters of dementia suffers go undiagnosed. *Daily Telegraph*, 1 March. Available at: www.telegraph.co.uk/health/healthnews/8353257/Up-to-three-quarters-of-dementia-sufferers-undiagnosed.html

Adams, T (2008) *Dementia care nursing: promoting well-being in people with dementia and their families.* Basingstoke: Palgrave Macmillan.

ADI (Alzheimer's Disease International) (2009) *Global prevalence of dementia.* Available at: www.alz.co.uk/research/files/WorldAlzheimerReport.pdf.

ADI (2010) *Global prevalence of dementia.* Available at www.alz.co.uk/research/files/WorldAlzheimer Report2010.pdf.

ADI (2011) *Common symptoms of dementia.* Available at: www.alz.co.uk/about-dementia.

Age Concern (2007) Delirium; Stop it, Treat it, Stop it. In *Toolkit for nursing homes.* Available at: www.nmhdu.org.uk/silo/files/lets-respect-toolkit-for-care-homes-pdf.

Alagiakrishnan, K (2008) Ethnic elderly with dementia: overcoming the cultural barriers to their care. *Canadian Family Physician*, 54, April: 521–22.

Alzheimer's Society (2008a) *Dementia: out of the shadows.* London: Alzheimer's Society. Available at: http://alzheimers.org.uk/site/scripts/download_info.php?fileID=454.

Alzheimer's Society (2008b) *Dementia UK.* London: Alzheimer's Society. Available at: http://alzheimers.org.uk/site/scripts/download_info.php?fileID=2.

Alzheimer's Society (2009) *Counting the cost: caring for people with dementia on hospital wards.* Available at: http://alzheimers.org.uk/site/scripts/download_info.php?fileID=787.

Alzheimer's Society (2010a) *Alzheimer's Society comment on new dementia prevalence statistics.* Available at: www.alzheimers.org.uk/site/scripts/press_article.php?pressReleaseID=398.

Alzheimer's Society (2010b) *Fact sheets for each of the more common type of dementia.* Available at: http://alzheimers.org.uk/factsheets.

Alzheimer's Society (2011) *Drug treatments for Alzheimer's disease.* Available at: www.alzheimers.org.uk/site/scripts/documents_info.php?documentID=147.

APA (American Psychiatric Association) 2011. *DSM-IV-TR: the current manual.* Available at: www.psych.org/MainMenu/Research/DSMIV/DSMIVTR.aspx.

Audit Commission (2000) *Forget me not.* London: TSO.

Audit Commission (2002) *Forget me not.* London: TSO.

Baines, P (2008) Art therapy and dementia care, in Adams, T (ed) *Dementia care nursing: promoting well-being in people with dementia and their families.* Basingstoke: Palgrave Macmillan.

Barker, S (2007) *Vital notes for nurses: psychology.* Oxford: Blackwell Publishing.

Barker, S (2011) *Midwives' emotional care of women becoming mothers.* Newcastle-upon-Tyne: CSP.

Beauchamp, T L and Childress, J F (2001) *Principles of biomedical ethics*, 5th edition. New York: Oxford University Press.

Berk, L E (2008). *Exploring lifespan development.* London: Pearson, Allyn & Bacon.

Boise, L (2008). Ethnicity and the experience of dementia, in Downs, M and Bower, B (eds) *Excellence in dementia care: research into practice.* Maidenhead: McGraw Hill Open University Press: 52–70.

Brannelly, T (2008) Developing an ethical basis for relationship-centred and inclusive approaches towards dementia care nursing, in Adams, T (ed) *Dementia care nursing: promoting well-being in people with dementia and their families.* Basingstoke: Palgrave Macmillan: 243–60.

Brinich, P and Shelley, C (2002) *The self and personality structure.* Buckingham: Open University Press.

Brunnstrom, H, Gustafson, L, Passant, U and Englund, E (2009) Prevalence of dementia subtypes: a 30 year retrospective survey of neuropathological reports. *Archives of Gerontology and Geriatrics*, 49: 146–49.

Burger, J M (2011) *Introduction to personality*, international edition, 8th edition. Belmont: Wadsworth, Cengage Learning.

Cantley, C (2001) *A handbook of dementia care*. Buckingham: Open University Press.

Centre for Cultural Diversity and Aging (2011) *Dementia care*. Available at: www.culturaldiversity.com.au/practice-guides/dementia-care.

Cheston, R and Bender, M (1999) *Understanding dementia, the man with the worried eyes*. London: Jessica Kingsley Publishers.

Cox, S and Keady, J (1999) *Younger people with dementia: planning, practice and development*. London: Jessica Kingsley Publishers.

CQC (Care Quality Commission) (2011) *Dignity and nutrition inspection programme*. Available at: www.cqc.org.uk/sites/default/files/media/documents/20111007_dignity_and_nutrition_inspection_report_final_update.pdf.

Crowe, S (1999) Alcohol-related brain impairment, in Cox, S and Keady, J (eds) *Younger people with dementia: planning, practice and development*. London: Jessica Kingsley Publishers.

Daily Mail (2011) *Barbaric treatment that shames the NHS*. Daily Mail, 14 October. Available at: www.dailymail.co.uk/debate/article-2048899/Barbaric-treatment-elderly-shames-NHS.html.

Dementia UK (2011) *Carers' experiences*. Available at: http://www.dementiauk.org/what-we-do/uniting-carers/carers-experiences/

DeMuth, D H (2004) Another look at resilience: challenging the stereotype of aging. *Journal of Feminist Therapy*, 16 (4): 61–74.

DH (Department of Health) (1999) *National service framework for mental health*. Available at: www.dh.gov.uk/en/Publicationsandstatistics/Publications/PublicationsPolicyAndGuidance/DH_4009598.

DH (2000) *No secrets: guidance on developing and implementing multi-agency policies and procedures to protect vulnerable adults from abuse*. Available at: www.dh.gov.uk/en/Publicationsandstatistics/Publications/Publications PolicyAndGuidance/DH_4008486.

DH (2001a) *National service framework for older people*. London: TSO.

DH (2001b) *Essence of care*. London: TSO.

DH (2001c) *The Single Assessment Process: consultation papers and process*. London: TSO.

DH (2004) *Carers and Disabled Children Act 2000 and Carers (Equal Opportunities) Act 2004 combined policy guidance*. Available at: www.dh.gov.uk/en/Publicationsandstatistics/Publications/PublicationsPolicyAnd Guidance/DH_4118023.

DH (2005) Care Services Improvement Partnership: *Everybody's business – integrated mental health services for older adults: a service development guide*. London: TSO.

DH (2005/2007) *Mental Health Act – Mental Capacity Act*. Available at: www.legislation.gov.uk/ukpga/2007/12/contents.

DH (2006) Reviewing the Care Programme Approach: a consultation process. London: Department of Health.

DH (2009) *Living well with dementia: a National Dementia Strategy*. London: TSO.

DH (2010a) *Quality outcomes for people with dementia: building on the work of the National Dementia Strategy*. Available at: www.dh.gov.uk/en/publicationsandstatistics/publications/publicationsPolicyAndGuidance/DH_119827.

DH (2010b) *Equity and excellence: liberating the NHS*. London: Department of Health.

DH (2010c) *Transparency in outcomes: a framework for the NHS*. London: Department of Health.

DH (2010d) *Essence of care: benchmarks for respect and dignity*. Available at: www.dh.gov.uk/prod_consum_dh/groups/dh_digitalassets/@dh/@en/@ps/documents/digitalasset/dh_119966.pdf.

DH (2011a) *Common core principles for supporting people with dementia*. Available at: www.dh.gov.uk/prod_consum_dh/groups/dh_digitalassets/documents/digitalasset/dh_127587.pdf.

DH (2011b) *Service specification for dementia: memory service for early diagnosis and intervention*. Available at: http://dementia.dh.gov.uk/memory-assessment-service-specifications/.

DH (2011c) *Safeguarding adults: the role of health services*. Available at: www.dh.gov.uk/en/Publicationsand statistics/Publications/PublicationsPolicyAndGuidance/DH_124882.

Docherty, T (2011) Legal and ethical issues in mental health nursing, in Trenoweth, S, Docherty, T, Franks, J and Pearce, R *Nursing and mental health care: an introduction for all fields of practice*. Exeter: Learning Matters.

Downs, M (2000) Dementia in a socio-cultural context: an idea whose time has come. *Aging and Society*, 20: 369–75.

Downs, M and Bowers, B (2008) *Excellence in dementia care: research into practice*. Maidenhead: McGraw-Hill, Open University Press.

Draper, P and McSherry, W (2007) Culture, religion and spirituality, in Nemo, R, Aveyard, B and Heath, H (eds) *Older people and mental health nursing: a handbook of care*. Oxford: Blackwell Publishing: 115–21.

Du, Peng (2011) *The global burden of dementia worldwide*. IAGG/WHO/SFGG, 13–14 January, Geneva Switzerland.

Ebersole, P and Hess, P (1998) *Towards healthy aging: human needs and nursing response*, 5th edition. London: Mosby.

Ferri, C P, Prince, M K, Brayne, C, Brodaty, H, Frutiglioni, L, Ganguli, M, Hall, K, Hasegawa, K, Hendric, H, Huang, Y, Jorm, A, Mather, C, Menezes, P R, Rimmer, E and Scazfca, M (2005) Global prevalence of dementia: a Delphi consensus study. *Lancet*, 36: 2112–17.

Folstein, M F, Folstein, S E and McHugh, P R (1975) Mini mental state: a practical method for grading the cognitive state of patients for clinicians. *Journal of Psychiatric Research*, 12: 189–98.

Forbat, L (2008) Social policy and relationship-centred dementia nursing, in Adams, T (ed) *Dementia care nursing: promoting well-being in people with dementia and their families*. Basingstoke: Palgrave Macmillan: 227–242.

Foreman, M (1996) Nursing strategies for acute confusion in elders. *American Journal of Nursing*, 96 (4): 44–51.

Gallagher-Thompson, D, Haley, W, Guy, D, Rupert, M, Arguelles, T, Zeiss, L M, Long, C, Tennstedt, S and Ory, M (2003) Tailoring psychological interventions for ethnically diverse dementia caregivers. *Clinical Psychology: Science and Practice*, 10 (4): 423–38.

Gross, R (2001) *Psychology, the science of mind and behaviour*, 4th edition. London: Hodder & Stoughton.

Guardian (2011) Hospital staff 'lack skills to cope with dementia patients'. Guardian, 16 December.

Hall, C (2004) Young nurses 'too posh to wash'. *Telegraph*, 19 October. Available at: www.telegraph.co.uk/news/uknews/1461504/Young-nurses-too-posh-to-wash.html

Harvey, R J, Skelton-Robinson, M and Rosser, M N (2003) The prevalence and cause of dementia in people under the age of 65 years. *Journal of Neurology, Neurosurgery & Psychiatry*, 74: 1206–09.

Henry, M (2002) Descending into delirium. *American Journal of Nursing*, 102 (3): 49–56.

Hodge, S (2008) Dementia care nursing: the legal framework, in Adams, T (ed) *Dementia care nursing: promoting well-being in people with dementia and their families*. Basingstoke: Palgrave Macmillan: 260–78.

Hornby, S and Atkins, J (2000) *Collaborative care: interprofessional, interagency and interpersonal*. Oxford: Blackwell Publishing.

ILC (International Longevity Centre) Global Alliance (2010) *The globalisation of dementia: issues and responses*. Available at: www.ilcjapan.org/symposiumE/1010.html.

ILC Global Alliance (2011) *The European Dementia Research Agenda*. Available at: www.ilc-alliance.org/book/european-dementia-research-agenda.html.

Jamieson, S. (1999) HIV-related brain impairment, in Cox, S and Keady, J (eds) *Younger people with dementia: planning practice and development*. London: Jessica Kingsley Publishers.

Killick, J and Allen, K (2001) *Communication and the care of people with dementia*. Buckingham: Open University Press.

Kitwood, T (1993) Person and process in dementia. *International Journal of Geriatric Psychiatry*, 8: 40–56.

Kitwood, T (1997) *Dementia reconsidered, the person comes first*. Maidenhead: Open University Press.

Kitwood, T and Bredin, K (1992) Toward a theory of dementia: personhood and well being. *Aging and Society*, 12: 269–87.

Kolb, B and Whishaw, I Q (2006) *An introduction to brain and behaviour*, second edition. New York: Worth Publishers.

Lee, H and Adams, T (2011) *Creative approaches in dementia care*. Basingstoke: Palgrave.

Lefrancois, G R (1999) *The Lifespan*, sixth edition. London: Wadsworth Publishing Company.

MacKinlay, E B (2001) The spiritual dimension of caring: applying a model for spiritual tasks of aging. *Journal of Religious Gerontology*, 12 (3,4): 151–66.

MacKinlay, E B (2011) Creative processes to bring out expressions of spirituality: working with people who have dementia, in Lee, H and Adams, T (eds) *Creative approaches in dementia care.* Basingstoke: Palgrave Macmillan.

MCA (2005) *Mental Capacity Act 2005.* Available at: www.legislation.gov.uk/ukpga/2005/9/contents.

MCA (2007) *Code of Practice, Mental Capacity Act 2005.* Available at: www3.imperial.ac.uk/pls/portallive/docs/1/51771696.PDF.

McCance, T V, McKenna, H P and Boore, J R P (1999) Caring: theoretical perspectives of relevance to nursing. *Journal of Advanced Nursing,* 30 (6), 1388–95.

MHA (2007) Mental Health Act 2007. Available at: www.legislation.gov.uk/ukpga/2007/12/contents.

Mioshi, E, Dawson, K, Mitchell, J, Arnold, R and Hodges, R J (2006) The Addenbrooke's Cognitive Examination Revised (ACE-R); a brief cognitive test battery for dementia screening. *International Journal of Geriatric Screening,* 21: 1078–85.

Mitsuyama, Y and Inoue, T (2009) Clinical entity of frontotemporal dementia with motor neurone disease. *Neuropathology,* 29: 649–54.

Morris, G and Morris, J (2010) *The dementia care workbook.* Maidenhead: McGraw-Hill, Open University Press.

Mutsatsa, S (2011) *Medicines management in mental health nursing: transforming nursing practice.* Exeter: Learning Matters.

Napoles, A M, Chadiha, L, Eversley, R and Moreno-John, G (2010) Developing culturally sensitive dementia caregiver interventions: are we there yet? *American Journal of Alzheimer's Disease and other Dementias,* 25 (5): 389–406.

Nath, A, Schiess, S, Venkatesan, A, Rumbaugh, J, Sacktor, N and Mcarthur, J (2008) Evolution of HIV dementia with HIV infection. *International Review of Psychiatry,* 20 (1): 25–31.

NCPC (National Council for Palliative Care) (2012) *Palliative care explained.* Available at: www.ncpc.org.uk/site/professionals/explained.

NHS (2012) *National End of life Care Programme.* Available at: www.endoflifecareforadults.nhs.uk/strategy.

NICE (National Institute for Health and Clinical Excellence) (2010) *Dementia quality standards.* Available at: www.nice.org.uk/aboutnice/qualitystandards/dementia/dementiaqualitystandard.jsp.

NICE (2011a) *About NICE guidance.* Available at: http://guidance.nice.org.uk/.

NICE (2011b) *Dementia pathway.* Available at: http://pathways.nice.org.uk/pathways/dementia.

NICE and SCIE (Social Care Institute for Excellence) (2006) *Dementia: supporting people with dementia and their carers in health and social care* (CG42). London: TSO. Available at: www.nice.org.uk/nicemedia/pdf/CG042NICEGuideline.pdf.

NMC (2010a) *Standards for pre-registration nursing education.* Available at: http://standards.nmc-uk.org.

NMC (2010b) *Raising and escalating concerns guidance.* Available at: www.nmc-uk.org/Nurses-and-midwives/Raising-and-escalating-concerns/.

NMC (2011) *The code: standards of conduct, performance and ethics for nurses and midwives.* Available at: www.nmc-uk.org/Nurses-and-midwives/The-code/The-code-in-full/.

Nolan, M R, Davies, S, Brown, J, Keady, J and Nolan, J (2004) Beyond 'person centred' care: a new vision for gerontological nursing. *International Journal of Older People Nursing in association with Journal of Clinical Nursing,* 13 (3a): 45–53.

Nuffield Council on Bioethics (2009) *Dementia: ethical issues.* Cambridge: Cambridge Publishers.

ONS (Office for National Statistics) (2011) *Deaths registered in England and Wales in 2010 by cause.* Available at: www.ons.gov.uk/ons/dcp171778_239518.pdf.

Parker, C and Philp, I (2004) Screening for cognitive impairment among older people in black and minority ethnic groups. *Age and Aging,* 33: 447–52.

Parker, M (2001) *Nursing theories and nursing practice.* Philadelphia PA: F A Davis Company.

Parry, J and Weiyuan, C (2011) Looming dementia epidemic in Asia. *Bulletin of the World Health Organization,* 89: 166–67.

Patient.co.uk (2012) *Memory loss and dementia, related resources.* Available at: www.patient.co.uk/health/Memory-Loss-and-Dementia/professional.

Phillips, M (2011) The real reason our hospitals are a disgrace. *Mail online*, 17 October. Available at: www.dailymail.co.uk/debate/article-2049906/How-feminism-nurses-grand-care.html?ITO=1490.

Pratchett, T (2008) Terry Pratchett: I'm slipping away a bit at a time . . . and all I can do is watch it happen. *Daily Mail*, 7 October. Available at: www.dailymail.co.uk/health/article-1070673/Terry-Pratchett-Im-slipping-away-bit-time—I-watch-happen.html.

RCN (Royal College of Nursing) (2008) *Dignity*. Available at: www.rcn.org.uk/newsevents/campaigns/dignity.

RCP (Royal College of Physicians) (2007) *Clinical guidelines for the assessment of pain in older people*. Available at: www.bgs.org.uk/Publications/Clinical%20Guidelines/pain%20concise%20guidelines%20WEB.pdf.

RCPsych (Royal College of Psychiatrists) (2011a) *Report of the National Audit of Dementia Care in General Hospitals 2011*. Available at: www.rcpsych.ac.uk/pdf/NATIONAL%20REPORT%20-%20Exec%20Summary%202911.pdf.

RCPsych (2011b) *Reform of mental health legislation*. Available at: www.rcpsych.ac.uk/policy-1/parliamentand publicaffairs/aboutourparliamentarywork/westminster/mhbill.aspx.

Rewston, C and Moniz-Cook, E (2008) Understanding and alleviating emotional distress, in Downs, M and Bowers, B (eds) *Excellence in dementia care: research into practice*. Maidenhead: McGraw-Hill, Open University Press: 249–63.

Robertson-Gillam, K (2011) Music therapy in dementia care, in Lee, H and Adams, T (eds) *Creative approaches in dementia care*. Basingstoke: Palgrave: 91–109.

Rogers, C R (1951) *Client centred therapy*. London: Constable.

Roper, N, Logan, W and Tierney, A (1980) *The elements of nursing*, 1st edition. Edinburgh: Churchill Livingstone.

Rothman, B K (2000) *Recreating motherhood*. New York: WW Norton & Company.

SfC (Skills for Care) and SfH (Skills for Health) (2011) *Common and core principles for supporting people with dementia*. Available at: www.dh.gov.uk/en/Publicationsandstatistics/Publications/PublicationsPolicy AndGuidance/DH_127442.

Stephan, B and Brayne, C (2008) Prevalence and projections of dementia, in Downs, M and Bowers, B (eds) *Excellence in dementia care, research into practice*. Maidenhead: McGraw-Hill, Open University Press: 9–35.

Stuart-Hamilton, I (2000) *The psychology of aging: an introduction*, 3rd edition. London: Jessica Kingsley Publishers.

Todres, L, Galvin, K T and Holloway, I (2009) The humanization of healthcare: a value framework for qualitative research. *International Journal of Qualitative Studies on Health and Well-being*, 4: 66–77.

Verity, J and Lee, H (2011) Reigniting the human spirit, in Lee, H and Adams, T (eds) *Creative approaches in dementia care*. Basingstoke: Palgrave: 16–32.

Wade, D T and Halligan, P W (2004) Do biomedical models of illness make for good health care systems? *BMJ*, 329 (7479: 1398).

WHO (World Health Organization) (2010) *International classification of diseases – 10*. Available at: http://apps.who.int/classifications/icd10/browse/2010/en#/F00-F09.

WHO (2012) *Definition of palliative care*. Available at: www.who.int/cancer/palliative/definition/en/.

Index